Brain Imaging:
An Introduction

Brain Imaging:
An Introduction

John R. Bradshaw
BA, MB, BCh, DMRD, FRCR, FRCP(C)
Consultant Neuroradiologist, Frenchay Hospital, Bristol

Wright
London   Boston   Singapore   Sydney   Toronto   Wellington

First published, 1989

© **Butterworth & Co. (Publishers) Ltd, 1989**

British Library Cataloguing in Publication Data

Bradshaw, John R.
   Brain imaging: an introduction.
   1.   Brain—Diseases—Diagnosis
   2.   Brain—Radiography
   3.   Diagnostic imaging
   I. Title
   616.8'04754   RC386.6.R3

   ISBN 0-7236-0596-3

Library of Congress Cataloging-in-Publication Data

   Brain imaging: an introduction
   Bradshaw, John R.
      p.   cm.
   Bibliography: p.
   Includes indexes.
   ISBN 0-7236-0596-3
   1. Brain—Imaging.
   2. Brain—Diseases—Diagnosis.
   I. Title.
   [DNLM: 1. Brain—radiography.
   2. Brain—radionuclide imaging.
   3. Brain Diseases—diagnosis.
   4. Nuclear Magnetic Resonance—methods.
   5. Ultrasonic Diagnosis—methods.
   WL 141 B812b]
   RC386.6.D52B73 1988
   616.8'04754—dc19

Photoset by Mid-County Press, London
Printed and bound in Great Britain by Butler and Tanner, Frome, Somerset

Preface

An accurate and definitive diagnosis is the cornerstone of all medical management. Nowhere is this more true than in diseases of the brain. Neuroradiology has been at the forefront of the drive to embrace and realize the full potential of new diagnostic techniques. The past 30 years have seen rapid advances in medical technology and these have been most visible in diagnostic radiology. Catheter arteriography, computed tomography and magnetic resonance imaging have all found their first footholds in the arena of brain diagnosis. Consequently, the approach to the diagnosis of brain disease has changed dramatically, particularly in the past 10 years. Furthermore, a new era of change has been ushered in with the recent arrival of magnetic resonance imaging. This has rapidly asserted itself as a vital element in the assessment of brain and spinal pathology.

As the range of possible techniques for brain diagnosis widens, the need for guidance as to which technique is most appropriate for a given problem has never been more acute. It is the purpose of this book to fill this need and to illustrate the diverse manifestations of brain disease as revealed by these techniques. The style and content of the book have been chosen to appeal to a wide variety of readers, including student and qualified radiologists, other clinicians of both consultant and junior status, nurses, radiographers, etc.

It would be impossible to mention individually the countless colleagues and institutions who have contributed illustrations for this book: I can only express my sincere thanks. However, specific mention must be made of: The Bristol MRI Centre, Dr Derek Kingsley (Queen Square Imaging Centre), Dr David Miller (MS Research Unit, National Hospital) and Dr Peter Cavanagh (Kerland Institute) who have generously permitted reproduction of MRI scans of patients under their care. Dr Ian Ferguson, Mr Hugh Coakham, Dr Peter Jackson and Dr Tim Lewis, who have patiently guided my hand through the complexities of neurology, neurosurgery and magnetic resonance, deserve my special thanks. Any misconceptions that remain are mine alone.

Dr Gordon Thomson has provided a receptive ear and a breadth of experience that few could match. His friendship and enthusiasm have done much to sustain me.

The quality of the images is a tribute to the many radiographers and others who continue to pursue high standards in the face of an increasing range and complexity of the techniques with which they work.

Finally, it would have been impossible for me to complete this book without the patient and indulgent support of my wife. In addition to typing the many drafts, she has brought further expertise to my faltering syntax.

May 1987   JRB

Contents

List of abbreviations

AP	anteroposterior
AVM	arteriovenous malformation
CPA	cerebellopontine angle
CSF	cerebrospinal fluid
CT	computerized axial tomography
FID	free induction decay
IR	inversion recovery
MRI	magnetic resonance imaging
NMR	nuclear magnetic resonance
PA	posteroanterior
RF	radiofrequency
SAH	subarachnoid haemorrhage
SE	spin-echo
SR	saturation recovery
TE	time to echo
TI	time to inversion
TIA	transient ischaemic attack
TR	repetition time
US	ultrasound

Introduction

Format

The book is divided into two parts. The first describes each of the current diagnostic techniques, with indications for their use and an outline of the basic anatomy and pathology that can be revealed by them. In the second part, brain disease as revealed by these techniques is handled in a problem-orientated way. Consequently, instead of traditional chapters dealing with tumours, infection, vascular disorders and so on, the material is organized according to the patient's presenting features—headaches, fits, weakness, etc. This format seems more practical and is ideally suited to an approach which emphasizes a logical choice of diagnostic technique.

Within Part II, each clinical presentation starts with a summary of the symptoms and an outline of the common causes. This is followed by a series of case presentations illustrating those causative conditions that can be diagnosed by contemporary diagnostic imaging. The 100 case presentations are designed to illustrate the many clinical, anatomical and pathological concepts involved, together with the application and interpretation of the most appropriate imaging techniques. The case presentations can also be used as self-examination exercises by covering up the right-hand page and studying the images and information on the left side. Having made a diagnosis from these data, the reader's decision can be compared with the analysis on the right.

For those readers who need to study a pathological subject as a whole, say 'infarction' or hydrocephalus', then the pathology index on p. 243 shows where all the appropriate cases can be found. The final pages also contain a complete index and a list of suggested further reading.

Throughout the book a basic understanding of simple clinical, anatomical and pathological terms is assumed. Detailed technical descriptions have been studiously avoided as such information is largely unnecessary in a work at this level. An exception has been made in the case of MRI, however. This technique will be so unfamiliar to most readers, and the information contained in its images so complex, that a more detailed account of its physical and biological features is indicated.

Throughout the book left and right are represented according to established conventions. On frontal films, and coronal images such as CT, ultrasound and MRI, the patient appears to face the reader with the patient's left on the reader's right. On axial images (CT and MRI) the patient's left is on the reader's left. Contrast-enhanced CT images are marked '[+C]'.

Imaging techniques in brain diagnosis

Since CT scanning became established as the mainstay of brain imaging there has been a tendency to diminish the role of plain radiographs of the skull. This is a mistake. Vital basic information is often seen only on plain films and may be very difficult to see by other imaging techniques. Evidence of raised intracranial pressure, mild pituitary fossa enlargement, fractures and bone erosion or sclerosis are crucial data in the diagnosis of brain disease and often need to be excluded with plain films before a final diagnosis can be reached on other modalities. In addition, a chest radiograph should be obtained on every patient on whom neuroimaging is being undertaken.

Angiography is usually required for a full assessment of vascular lesions, particularly if surgery may be an appropriate element in management. Angiography may also be needed to arrive at a final diagnosis of certain tumours. This technique is not without its risks, and its use should only be considered when the additional information is likely to influence the patient's management significantly. Furthermore, it should not normally be undertaken without a preceding CT scan.

Isotope scanning is a sensitive method for the detection of brain lesions but has limited value in defining what such lesions might be. Its role has diminished considerably in recent years.

Air encephalography and ventriculography are now practically obsolete in countries where CT scanning is readily available. They are not covered in this book.

Diagnostic ultrasound has considerable value as a screening test for hydrocephalus or haemorrhage in the first year of life. It has found an important place in neonatal units as a preliminary to, or substitute for, further evaluation.

CT scanning has, understandably, assumed the role of the principal diagnostic technique in brain diagnosis. It has some important limitations and must be used intelligently with a full appreciation of its strengths and weaknesses.

Magnetic resonance imaging is the most recent image technique to become available. Although it has now been available for 10 years, much technical and clinical research will still be required before its full potential is established. This is mostly because it provides a much wider range of information than any of the other techniques, and the value of some measurements has yet to be established. Nevertheless, its worth in the assessment of white matter disease and posterior fossa lesions can no longer be disputed.

More detailed discussion of the indications for these techniques is included in the specific descriptions that follow for each imaging modality. The question of choosing the most appropriate techniques for the investigation of specific clincal problems is discussed in the various section introductions in Part II.

All imaging techniques have their advantages and disadvantages, not the least of which may be the risk to the patient, cost or limited availability. A clear understanding of the most effective and efficient use of these resources is the least we owe our patients.

Part I—The Techniques

Plain skull radiographs

Plain radiographs of the skull remain the most basic form of imaging for brain disorders. The skull frequently reflects the state of the brain contained within it, and in these days of sophisticated high-technology imaging techniques the value of plain films must not be underestimated or forgotten. Even techniques such as CT scanning or MRI may not show vault fractures, early enlargement of the pituitary fossa or evidence of raised intracranial pressure, etc. These and other signs are readily detected on plain skull radiographs however, and their presence may have a crucial impact on the patient's management. In this author's opinion, use of the more sophisticated techniques without at least some accompanying basic plain skull radiographs is unwise.

In the following pages the techniques and anatomy of the four most commonly used basic skull projections are described. This is followed by a selection of special views of various parts of the skull. Then follows a selection on normal variants, such as falx calcification and the like, commonly seen on skull films. Finally, a series of 22 illustrations is included, depicting basic pathological processes and particularly skull lesions that will not be illustrated under the various headings in Part II. This is necessary, since such conditions may give rise to neurological symptoms that are not primarily due to brain lesions or they may invade the cranial contents.

Technique

Plain skull radiographs can be obtained on quite basic X-ray equipment and with average radiographic skills. The best and most diagnostic films, however, are obtained by experienced staff using specially designed skull equipment. The four basic projections when properly taken and processed provide a wealth of information about the state of a patient's skull and, to a lesser extent, its contents. As a minimum, a lateral projection should be obtained. Four views will be more helpful, however, and the special views on pp. 4 and 5 provide additional detailed information about certain areas that are not well shown on the standard projections.

All skull films suffer from overlap. That is, many structures are projected on top of each other. The various projections help to unravel these bony features so that they can be properly assessed for any changes present. Detailed descriptions of the radiographic techniques are beyond the scope of this book.

Anatomy and pathology

Plain radiographs of the skull are primarily intended to reflect the various different densities in the bones of the skull, the cranial cavity and other adjacent structures. Bony structures are shown as white areas, the degree of 'whiteness' reflecting the thickness and mineralization of the area under consideration. Black areas are seen where normal air-filled structures are present, e.g., paranasal sinuses. Intracranial air and fractures show 'black' areas in regions where these would not be expected. Increased or decreased bony density may be part of a generalized process, or the result of some focal pathology. Under normal circumstances the two sides of the skull are symmetrical and this fact provides a useful comparison for suspected abnormalities on frontal projections. Certain normal and abnormal intracranial structures calcify, and when this is sufficiently dense it can be seen on plain films as a density similar to bone.

1

The lateral skull radiograph

This view (*Figure 1*) is obtained by directing an X-ray beam sideways at the skull, centring the beam 4 cm above the external auditory meatus. The film is placed on the opposite side of the head. This is a particularly useful projection, the only serious areas of overlap being in the petrous and facial bones. The pituitary fossa and vault are particularly well shown. The vault varies in thickness and shows some variation in density; this is often very prominent in children (convolutional markings).

A horizontal beam is often used to demonstrate air-fluid levels.

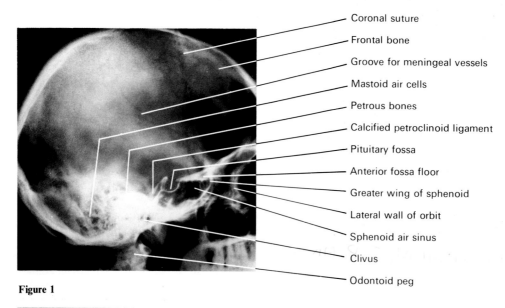

Coronal suture
Frontal bone
Groove for meningeal vessels
Mastoid air cells
Petrous bones
Calcified petroclinoid ligament
Pituitary fossa
Anterior fossa floor
Greater wing of sphenoid
Lateral wall of orbit
Sphenoid air sinus
Clivus
Odontoid peg

Figure 1

The PA 20° radiograph

This view (*Figure 2*) is obtained with the patient's face against the film and the X-ray beam entering the skull from behind (posteroanterior) in the midline at an angle of 20° to the canthomeatal line. This view provides good visualization of the vault, frontal and ethmoidal sinuses, orbital contents and sphenoid wings. The floor of the pituitary fossa can also be seen. The petrous bones are obscured, being projected over the maxillary antra.

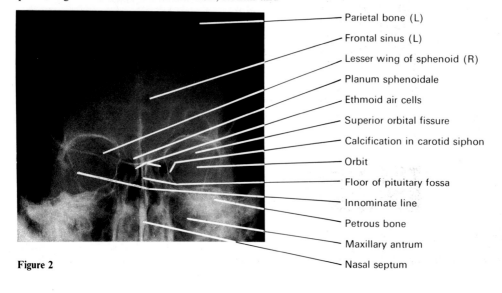

Parietal bone (L)
Frontal sinus (L)
Lesser wing of sphenoid (R)
Planum sphenoidale
Ethmoid air cells
Superior orbital fissure
Calcification in carotid siphon
Orbit
Floor of pituitary fossa
Innominate line
Petrous bone
Maxillary antrum
Nasal septum

Figure 2

Towne's projection (half-axial) AP

This projection (*Figure 3*) is obtained with the occiput against the film, while the X-ray beam is centred in the midline and angled 30° to the canthomeatal line. This view shows the occipital bone well, together with the petrous bones and foramen magnum. Anterior structures are projected downwards and obscured. The pineal gland is often calcified, as in this case.

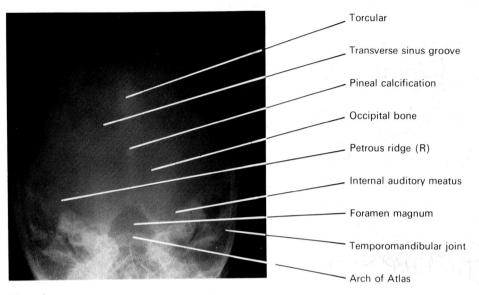

Torcular

Transverse sinus groove

Pineal calcification

Occipital bone

Petrous ridge (R)

Internal auditory meatus

Foramen magnum

Temporomandibular joint

Arch of Atlas

Figure 3

The base projection (submentovertical)

This view (*Figure 4*) requires considerable cooperation on the part of the patient as the neck must be fully extended. The film is placed against the skull vertex and the X-ray beam is then directed upwards between the angles of the mandible and at right angles to the film. This view, when correctly taken, provides an excellent view of the skull base, especially the foraminae, bony canals, petrous bones and paranasal sinuses. The occipital area, vault and frontal bones are mostly obscured.

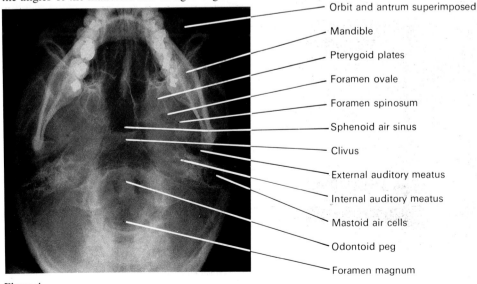

Orbit and antrum superimposed

Mandible

Pterygoid plates

Foramen ovale

Foramen spinosum

Sphenoid air sinus

Clivus

External auditory meatus

Internal auditory meatus

Mastoid air cells

Odontoid peg

Foramen magnum

Figure 4

The pituitary fossa

These projections (*Figures 5, 6*) are conventional views of the pituitary fossa but taken with a coned focal beam. Similar quality can be achieved on full skull radiographs if careful attention is given to centring and exposure. They are included here to facilitate anatomical demonstration.

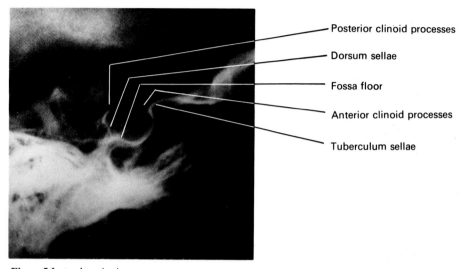

Posterior clinoid processes

Dorsum sellae

Fossa floor

Anterior clinoid processes

Tuberculum sellae

Figure 5 Lateral projection

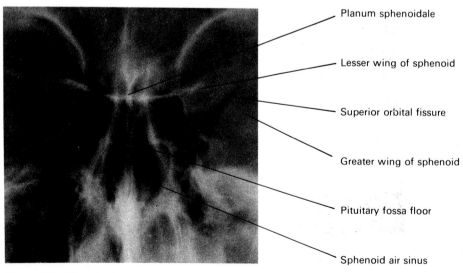

Planum sphenoidale

Lesser wing of sphenoid

Superior orbital fissure

Greater wing of sphenoid

Pituitary fossa floor

Sphenoid air sinus

Figure 6 PA 20° projection

Oblique projections of optic foramen/mastoid bone

Figure 7 is a useful specialized projection taken obliquely along the optic nerve canal. Each orbit is visualized separately (Ruggiero's method). This view is required because the canal runs obliquely to the conventional projections and is consequently obscured. The canal is seen end on. *Figure 8* is an oblique projection to show the mastoid air cells, external auditory meatus and temporomandibular joint.

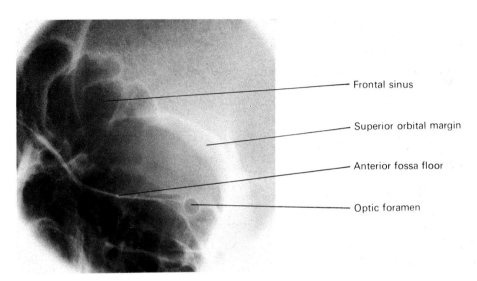

Frontal sinus

Superior orbital margin

Anterior fossa floor

Optic foramen

Figure 7

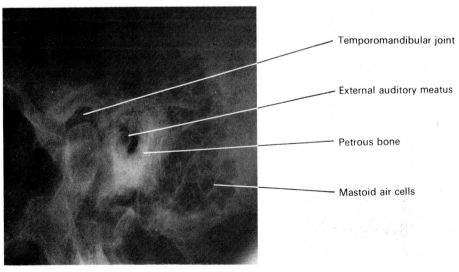

Temporomandibular joint

External auditory meatus

Petrous bone

Mastoid air cells

Figure 8

Stenver's projection

Stenver's projection (*Figure 9*) is an oblique view designed to align the petrous bone parallel to the film. This overcomes some of the problems encountered on conventional projections in visualizing this bone and its constituent structures.

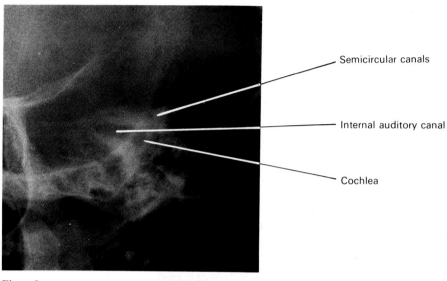

Semicircular canals

Internal auditory canal

Cochlea

Figure 9

Water's projection (*occipitomental*)

Water's projection (*Figure 10*) uses an angulation of the beam and head to show the maxillary antra clearly without overlap of the petrous bones. The orbits and zygomas are also well shown.

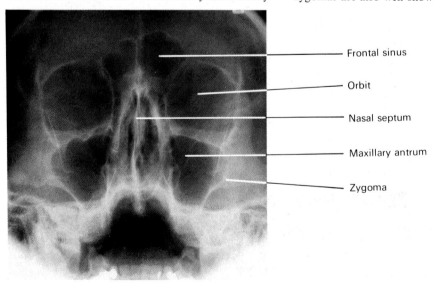

Frontal sinus

Orbit

Nasal septum

Maxillary antrum

Zygoma

Figure 10

Physiological intracranial calcification

Figure 11 shows a calcified pineal gland in the lateral projection. Because of its strategic midline position at the posterior aspect of the third ventricle, it can provide a useful marker for displacement of internal brain anatomy. When the calcified area is more than 1 cm in diameter a pineal tumour should be suspected. (*See* Case 11.)

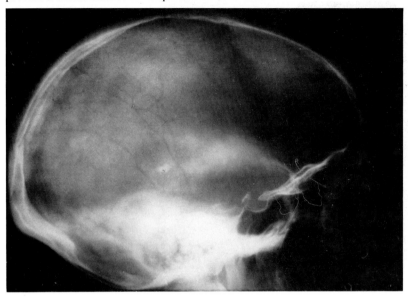

Figure 11

Figure 12 shows calcification in the choroid plexus. This is usually seen in the trigone region of the lateral ventricles. When the lateral view is straight, the calcification on the two sides is superimposed.

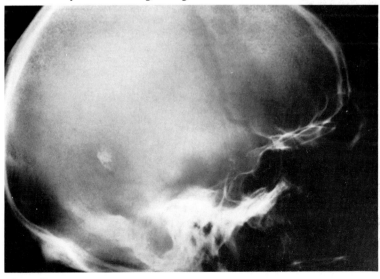

Figure 12

Figure 13 is a Towne's projection showing physiological calcification of the choroid plexus bilaterally (same case as *Figure 12*). The symmetry may be helpful as one trigone can be displaced by adjacent masses.

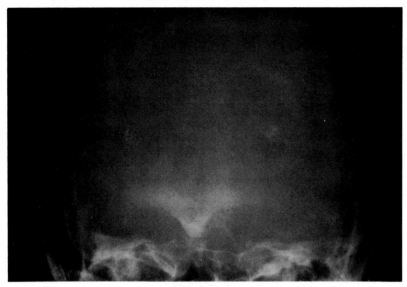

Figure 13

Figure 14 is a PA 20° projection showing midline calcification. This is located in the falx and appears this dense because it is seen end on. Only large masses are capable of causing shift of the falx. Calcification is quite common in the dura and may also be seen in the tentorium, over the convexity, or in the petroclinoid ligaments (*see Figure 1*).

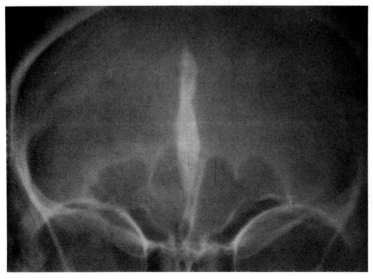

Figure 14

Occipital defects

Figure 15 shows a not uncommon normal variant with a 'bubbly' defect in the occipital bone. This is usually close to the midline and is variously ascribed to 'glial' rests or venous structures. It should not be mistaken for pathology.

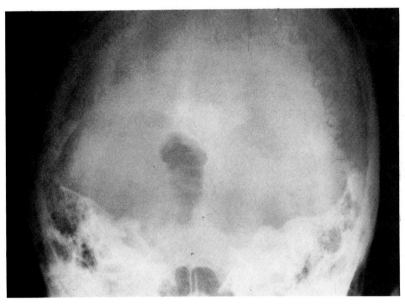

Figure 15

Carotid siphon calcification

Figure 16 shows serpiginous parallel lines of calcification superimposed on the pituitary fossa (arrow). This is due to atheroma in the carotid siphon and is common in older patients. In the PA 20° projection it can be seen as two rings of calcification outlining the vessel wall and lying on either side of the pituitary fossa floor (*see Figure 2*).

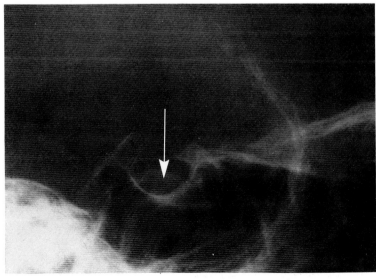

Figure 16

The infant skull

During the first 2 years of life the skull of a child is very different to that of an adult. This is because the sutures are very wide but not serrated at birth, and the fontanelles are still open (*Figures 17 and 18*). These margins between the vault bones gradually narrow until, at about 2 years, the overall appearance is very similar to that of an adult. Normally the sutures finally fuse during late teens.

Other features seen at various stages in the development of the skull include: convolutional impressions (2–14 years) on the inner table of the vault; gaps in the skull base at points where fusion of the various bones has yet to occur (synchondroses); metopic and mendosal sutures. More detailed accounts of the normal paediatric skull can be found in specialized texts.

The sinuses and mastoids are poorly pneumatized at birth but grow steadily in size and extent until adult life is reached.

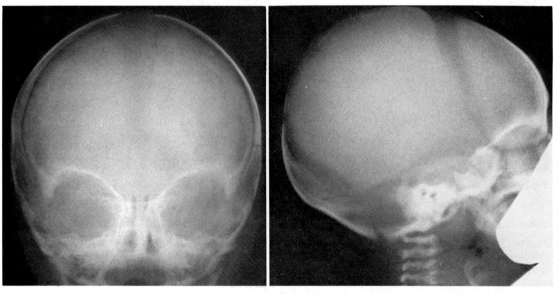

Figure 17   Figure 18

Raised intracranial pressure (child)

Figure 19 is a Towne's projection of the skull of a child aged 10 years. The lambdoid and sagittal sutures are seen to be separated with marked serration. This almost invariably indicates raised intracranial pressure. Other signs which may be seen include enlargement of the head, thinning of the bones of the vault and excessive convolutional markings.

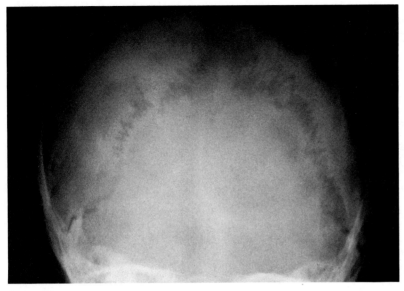

Figure 19

Lacunar skull/meningocele

Figure 20 shows an infant skull with multiple areas of severe bone thinning separated by ridges of bone. This defect of bone formation (also known as craniolacunia or luckenshadel) is often associated with midline defects as in this case, where a soft tissue mass is present in the occipital area due to a meningocele.

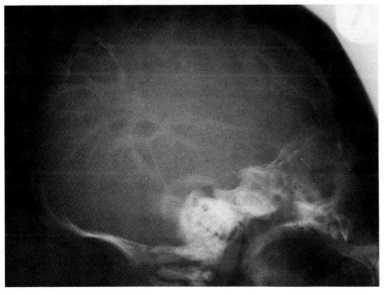

Figure 20

Craniostenosis/ventricular shunt

Premature fusion of the sutures can lead to raised intracranial pressure and deformity of the skull. Depending on which sutures are involved the skull may either grow vertically (turricephaly), as in this case where the coronal sutures have closed (*Figure 21*), or longitudinally (scaphocephaly) where the sagittal suture fuses prematurely. Other types also occur. The vault shows unduly prominent convolutional markings due to raised pressure. A ventricular shunt has been inserted and its metallic tip is clearly shown.

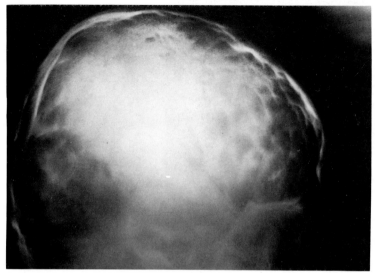

Figure 21

Platybasia

Platybasia is the name given to flattening of the skull base. This is measured using the basal angle (*Figure 22*). This angle is formed by lines joining the nasion and the tip of the clivus to the tuberculum sellae. Enlargement of this angle (normally 120–140°) is usually the result of a congenital deformity, but may be associated with other conditions causing softening of the base. It should not be confused with basilar invagination (*see* Cases 88 and 96).

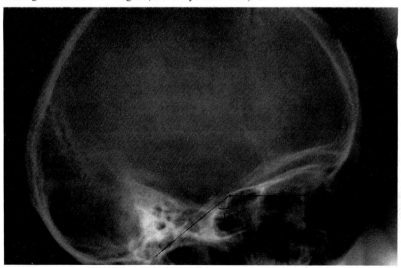

Figure 22

Midline shift

Figure 23 shows the calcified pineal gland to be displaced to the right-hand side from its normal midline location (arrow). This implies a mass effect in the left hemisphere with shift of midline structures—an important sign of intracranial pathology. Midline shift may also be seen on other imaging techniques. (Displacement of more than 3 mm is usually significant.)

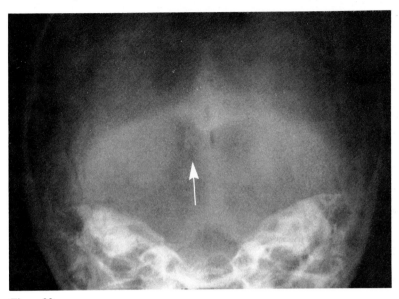

Figure 23

Intracranial calcification/raised intracranial pressure

Physiological calcification within the cranial cavity has been illustrated on previous pages. Many pathological processes produce calcification, including previous infection, vascular lesions and certain tumours. The pattern of calcification may be diagnostic (*see* Case 54). In the example in *Figure 24* a tumour in the parietal area is calcified and there is associated raised intracranial pressure. In adults this is manifested as erosion of the pituitary fossa floor and dorsum sellae. This usually indicates raised pressure of at least 4 weeks' duration. These signs usually occur independently, of course.

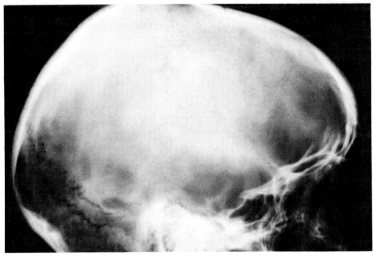

Figure 24

Fibrous dysplasia

This condition is characterized by patches of abnormal bone development showing well-defined reduced bone density with some thickening and modelling deformity. Facial bones are often involved as in the case in *Figure 25* (arrows). These lesions may present a 'ground-glass' texture. Involvement of the base may cause pressure on cranial nerves, or basilar invagination (Case 88).

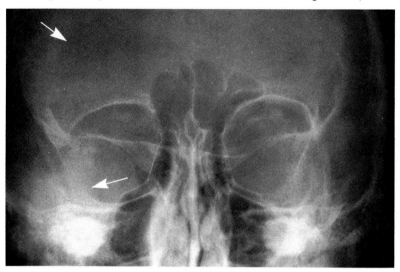

Figure 25

Metastatic disease

The bones of the skull are a common site for metastatic deposits. These may appear as areas of reduced density in the vault (*Figure 26*), or base (Case 60), or less commonly as ill-defined patches of sclerosis. Sclerotic deposits are usually the result of spread from tumours in the prostate or breast. Low density erosions may be confused with those of myeloma, which tend to be smaller and more diffuse than those of metastatic disease.

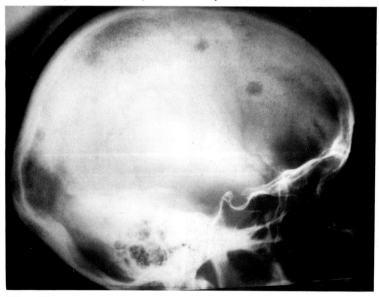

Figure 26

Haemangioma of vault

This uncommon tumour of blood vessels often produces a stippled area of rarefaction in the vault. Prominent vascular channels may run towards the lesion, as in the example in *Figure 27*. The appearances may be confused with a solitary metastatic or myeloma deposit. (An unrelated area of density in the vault is projected over the pituitary fossa.)

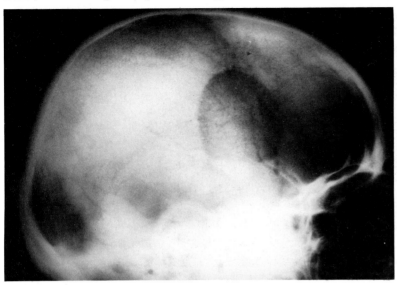

Figure 27

Epidermoid of vault

Developmental tumours are described more fully in Cases 4 and 33. They may also arise within bone. Dermoids characteristically arise at the outer angle of the orbit, and epidermoids in this location (*Figure 28*).

Contrast the sharply defined margin and thin sclerotic rim with the case illustrated in *Figure 27*. These lesions may extend from their bony location into the cranial cavity.

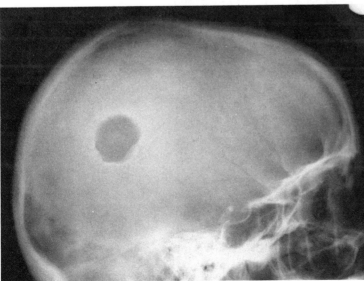

Figure 28

Burr hole/shunt

The skull radiograph in *Figure 29* shows a bone defect in the parietal area. The lesion is well-defined and without a sclerotic margin. Its location suggests it could be a surgical burr hole. These may be multiple and are used to aspirate haematomas, acquire biopsy material, or insert ventricular shunts. The metallic tip of the shunt tube can be seen more anteriorly.

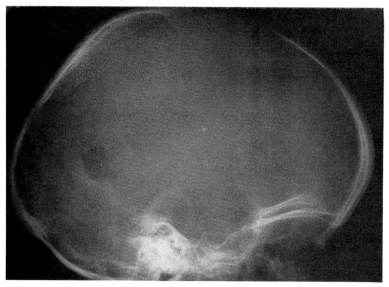

Figure 29

Craniotomy

Major access to the cranial cavity is acquired through a craniotomy. A flap of vault is elevated, often by cutting between a pattern of burr holes as illustrated here (*Figure 30*).

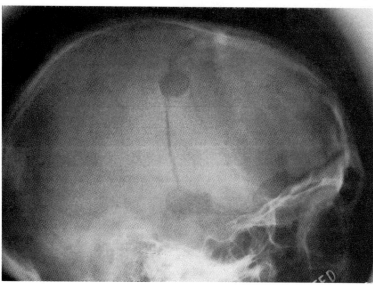

Figure 30

Osteoma of vault

The striking appearance of a well-defined area of dense bone extending outwards from the vault is due to an osteoma (*Figure 31*). This benign bony tumour may primarily grow outwards or inwards from the vault. It is quite harmless but local pressure may cause problems within the cranial cavity or in the scalp. This tumour is also commonly found in the frontal sinus.

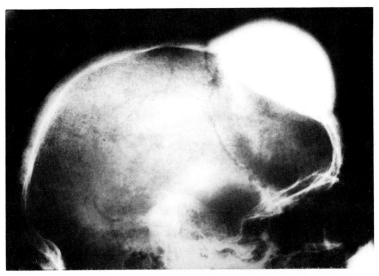

Figure 31

Hyperostosis of sphenoid wing (*meningioma*)

At the point of their attachment to the dura, meningiomas commonly provoke a hyperostosis or thickening of the underlying bone. A classical site is illustrated in *Figure 32*, where the left greater wing of sphenoid is involved causing the left orbit to appear denser than the right. There is coincidental opacification of the maxillary antra due to chronic sinus disease.

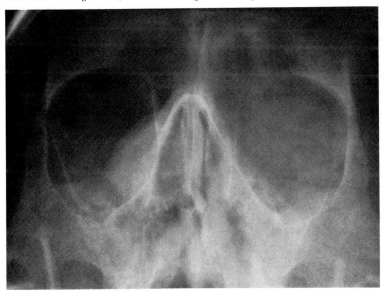

Figure 32

Skull fracture

Skull fractures by themselves are of limited significance, but they may be associated with other injuries of the intracranial contents such as extradural haematoma. Fractures that run into the skull base may breach the integrity of the dura and allow CSF to get out, or air or infection in. The Stenver's projection in *Figure 33* shows a typical fracture running vertically downwards from the lambdoid suture to the petrous bone. Note the different appearance of fracture (arrow) and suture.

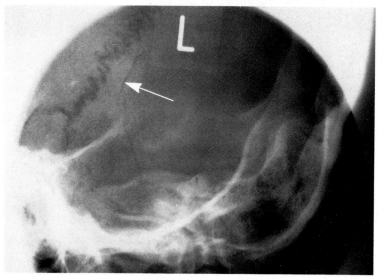

Figure 33

Intracranial air

The lateral skull film in *Figure 34* shows patches of very low density in the frontal area and over the pituitary fossa. These are due to pockets of air around the frontal lobes and within the ventricles. The intraventricular air lies within the temporal horns overlying the pituitary fossa. Such air may result from deliberate introduction during air studies, or surgery. In this case air has entered the cranial cavity through a fracture in the skull base.

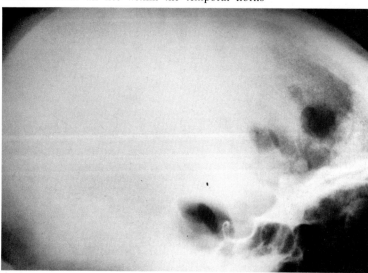

Figure 34

Leptomeningeal cyst

Figure 35 shows a long bone defect in the occipital area. This was associated with a soft tissue swelling and the patient had suffered a fracture at this site in childhood. This lesion is a 'growing' fracture due to a dural tear allowing pulsatile CSF to cause widening of the fracture and eventually varying degrees of local brain herniation.

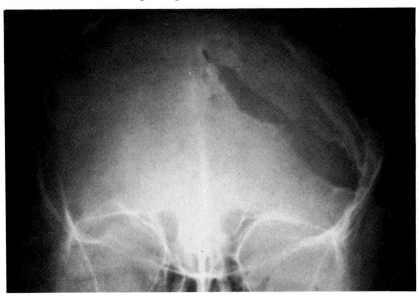

Figure 35

Optic nerve glioma

Figure 36 is a specific projection of the orbit (*see Figure 7*) and shows marked enlargement of the optic foramen. This structure carries the optic nerve and ophthalmic artery. When enlarged it usually indicates the presence of an optic nerve glioma (*see* Case 59).

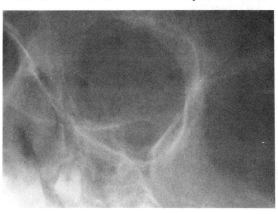

Figure 36

Basal ganglia calcification/parietal foraminae

Figure 37 shows prominent calcification on either side of the midline. Its configuration is quite symmetrical and when also visualized in the lateral film (*Figure 38*) its location is characteristic of the basal nuclei. A small amount of calcification is commonly seen in this location in older patients, especially on CT. When present to this degree it may indicate a disorder of parathyroid function. This patient also shows an unrelated developmental variant of the vault. Symmetrical rounded defects are present in the posterior parietal areas. During fetal life portions of the parietal bones are incomplete and these may persist into adult life. The defects slowly migrate posteriorly and are 1–2 cm in diameter. They are of no clinical significance but may be confused with pathological lesions.

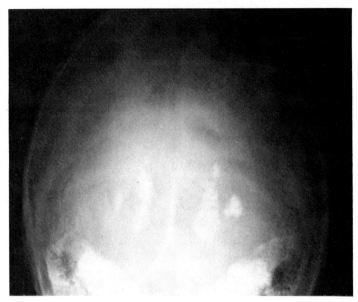

Figure 37

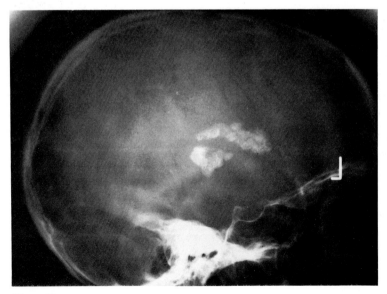

Figure 38

Enlargement of foramen ovale

Figure 39 is part of a base projection of the skull. The right foramen ovale (arrow) is considerably enlarged compared with the left side. A certain amount of asymmetry is normal but this degree of enlargement is excessive. The principal structure passing through this foramen is the mandibular division of the fifth cranial nerve and these changes are consistent with a neuroma of that nerve (*see also* Case 84).

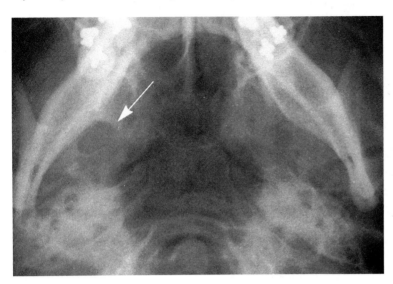

Figure 39

Plain-film tomography

Occasionally plain radiographs of the skull reveal an abnormal or suspicious area where the appearances are obscured by overlying structures or other features. The technique of plain-film tomography can be very effective in demonstrating the area under study to better advantage. This system employs controlled blurring of the image to remove much of the overlying features leaving only the structures in the desired plane, i.e., through the lesion, in focus. Special equipment is required for this purpose. CT scanning has replaced much of the need for plain-film tomography but several very useful applications remain.

The present indications for the use of plain-film tomography depend on the quality of CT available and time required for high-resolution CT studies. Even with good CT, the technique can provide very valuable and detailed information and assessment of calcifications and erosions in and above the skull base. Fractures of the base, petrous bones, cribriform plate, etc. are often best shown by this technique. Plain films of the pituitary fossa or internal auditory canals may be difficult to assess in cases where changes are borderline. Plain-film tomography may be very helpful in resolving such questions and provides data on which decisions can be made about the necessity to proceed to other techniques, such as CT and MRI. Some examples are shown below.

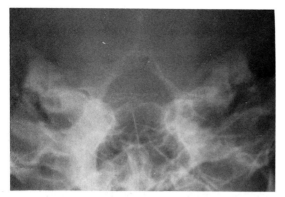

Figure 40

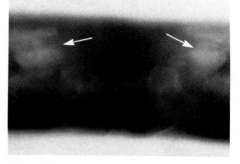

Figure 41

Figure 40 is a Towne's projection of the petrous bones in a patient with a clinical story suggestive of an acoustic neuroma. These lesions cause enlargement of the internal auditory canal which is not well visualized

here. *Figure 41* is a plain film tomograph centred through the internal canals which can now be clearly seen (arrows). They are both of equal size, making the diagnosis of acoustic tumour unlikely.

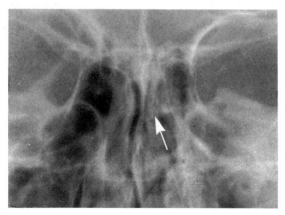

Figure 42

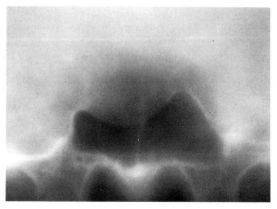

Figure 43

Figure 42 is a PA 20° projection in which the floor of the pituitary fossa (arrow) is poorly visualized (*see Figure 6*). The patient had symptoms suggesting endocrine dysfunction of pituitary origin. *Figure 43* shows the frontal tomograph through the pituitary

fossa on this patient. Now that overlying structures have been effaced by blurring, the profile of the floor is clearly visualized and the fossa is obviously deeply enlarged on the right (due to a tumour).

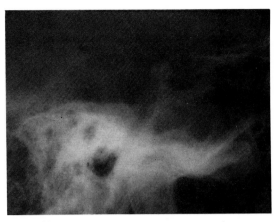

Figure 44

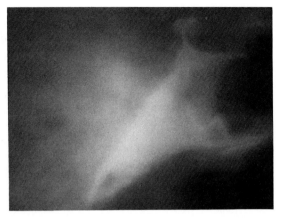

Figure 45

Figure 44 is a lateral projection in the region of the clivus and petrous bones. Because of overlapping bone density in these structures no useful detail is seen in this patient with brainstem signs and a mass in the anterior part of the posterior fossa on CT. *Figure 45*

shows the same area on tomography where the plane in focus is through the middle of the clivus. The clivus is unusually dense due to hyperostosis consistent with a diagnosis of meningioma. In this case tomography has further refined the data available on CT.

Radionuclide (isotope) brain scanning

Imaging of the brain using a radioactive isotope used to be a vital part of neuroradiological techniques. The advent of CT with its superior resolution and specificity has greatly reduced the importance of isotope scanning. When CT scanning is unavailable this technique still has a significant contribution to make, since it is quite sensitive to the detection of intracranial lesions. However, it is non-specific in determining what those lesions might be. When CT is available, the contribution of isotope scanning is limited to providing some back-up evidence for the presence of an early hemisphere lesion where CT is equivocal and to demonstrating abnormalities of the venous sinuses. Other specialized applications, such as detailed dynamic studies of the cerebral circulation and emission tomography, are beyond the scope of this book.

Technique

Routine isotope brain scanning is currently performed with an isotope called technetium-99m-labelled glucoheptonate. This has a half-life of 6 hours and the radiation dose to the patient is minimal. Nevertheless, isotope scanning should not be repeated unnecessarily, or used in children without good reason. A small dose of 15–20 mCi is given intravenously and after a delay of about 90 minutes to allow time for the isotope to circulate and become bound to the tissues, a series of scans is obtained in various projections using a rectilinear scanner or gamma camera.

Anatomy and pathology

The isotope is taken up by some normal structures, particularly the larger venous sinuses; the normal patterns are illustrated in *Figures 46–48*. Many brain lesions also take up the isotope, partly because of a disruption in the blood–brain barrier allowing the isotope to permeate into the tissue locally and accumulate there. Uptake is also due to increased vascularity and local changes in the distribution of water and other molecules in the affected tissues. The pattern of uptake, however, is not specific and most lesions produce rather similar appearances. Isotope imaging is quite sensitive and early lesions often show uptake even when CT is still equivocal for a definite lesion.

Normal isotope scans

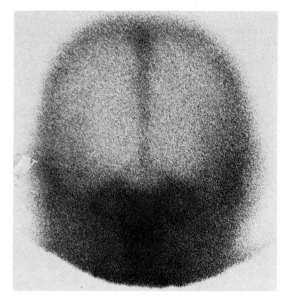

Figure 46

Figure 46 shows a normal anterior scan. High uptake due to vascularity in the skull base and neck muscles is normal and lesions close to this area may be obscured. A thin band of uptake is seen outlining the vault and a vertical band is due to isotope in the superior sagittal sinus anteriorly. The cerebral hemispheres show a uniform low uptake.

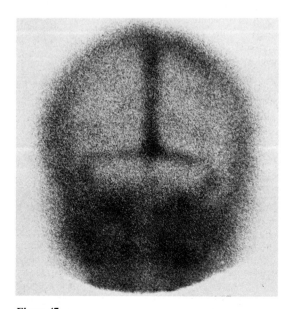

Figure 47

Figure 47 is of a normal posterior scan. The appearances are similar to the anterior view except that here the confluence of venous sinuses at the torcula is clearly shown as a cruciform area of uptake. It is normal for one lateral sinus to be bigger than the other.

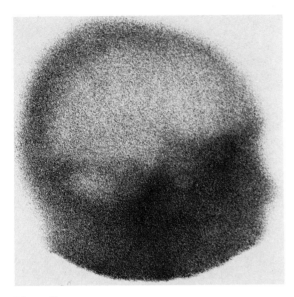

Figure 48

Figure 48 is of a normal lateral scan, the patient's face is on the right of the image. Scans of both sides of the brain are usually obtained. Similar areas of uptake are again seen but in this view the sagittal sinus lies on the vault uptake and is more intense posteriorly. The transverse sinus is also seen crossing the posterior fossa.

Cerebral ultrasound

Apart from some early work using a simple ultrasound probe to assess the position of midline structures, ultrasound was not used in the study of intracranial disease until the late seventies. Ultrasound waves at diagnostic frequencies do not really penetrate the vault and technical developments at that time led to the production of real-time sector scanning which could be used at the anterior fontanelle (a 'sonic window') to visualize intracranial structures. It rapidly became apparent that this technique could provide an excellent, convenient and inexpensive imaging system for brain disorders in neonates and young infants. Furthermore, the nature of the equipment meant that the examination could be performed at the bedside, often without sedation and with the minimum of disturbance for the patient. All these features were clearly advantageous in the management of young patients with suspected cerebral disorders. Although it is possible to obtain a sonic window elsewhere in the skull in certain situations, for practical purposes the examination is limited to those patients with a patent anterior fontanelle, i.e., up to the age of 9 months.

Indications

Ultrasound (US) assessment of intracranial disorders is now the first imaging technique of choice in neonates and young infants. In many instances the information is equal to that obtainable by CT and no further techniques will be required. The principal indications for US assessment are: increasing head size, dysmorphic features, myelomeningocele, inflammatory disease and asphyxia. Disorders that can be shown include hydrocephalus, intraventricular haemorrhage, subdural collections and focal lesions in the hemispheres, particularly cysts. Follow-up studies to monitor the progress of hydrocephalus, haemorrhage or other lesions are also particularly useful. Ultrasound is very effective in demonstrating these lesions and its accuracy equals CT in the demonstration of hydrocephalus, intraventricular haemorrhage and larger parenchymal lesions. It is not so accurate in the demonstration of smaller haemorrhages and parenchymal lesions, and in some subdural collections.

Technique

The examination requires a commercially available sector scanner with a transducer face narrow enough to provide proper contact at the limited area of the anterior fontanelle. Output around 5 MHz and a 90° field of vision are adequate. A series of scans in coronal and sagittal planes are obtained. Portable equipment enables the examination to be performed at the bedside or intensive care unit. Sedation is rarely required and there is no known hazard from cerebral ultrasound at diagnostic frequencies. Ultrasonic access to the intracranial cavity is also possible through other bone defects such as meningocele openings in the occiput, craniotomies, etc.

Normal ultrasound scans

Figure 49 shows a typical coronal scan of the brain of an infant aged 1 month. This scan shows the bodies of the lateral ventricles and the third ventricle clearly. On either side of these structures lie the basal nuclei. Below the third ventricle lies the suprasellar region.

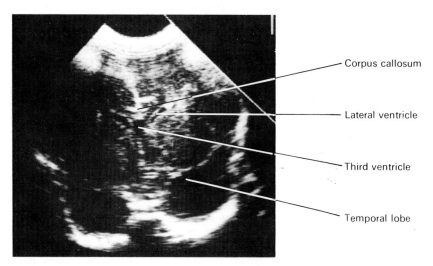

Corpus callosum

Lateral ventricle

Third ventricle

Temporal lobe

Figure 49

Figure 50 shows a normal parasagittal scan along the length of a lateral ventricle; the choroid plexus and temporal horn are demonstrated. The configuration of these structures on a scan will vary depending on the precise angulation of the probe.

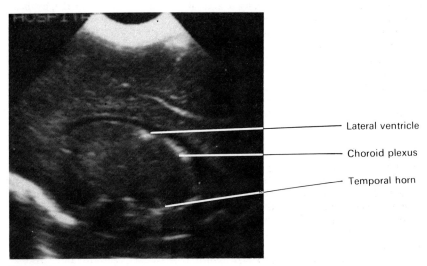

Lateral ventricle

Choroid plexus

Temporal horn

Figure 50

Cerebral angiography

Detailed radiographic studies of the cerebral vessels have been possible for many years. Until recently, such studies were obtained by injecting radio-opaque contrast medium into the carotid or vertebral arteries by direct puncture. More recently, catheters introduced by the femoral route are replacing direct puncture techniques. This transition and the newer, less toxic contrast media have greatly improved the safety and comfort of cerebral angiography. Prior to the advent of CT, angiography and air studies were the principal tools in the diagnosis of cerebral disease, especially tumours. However, CT scanning changed all that; air studies are now obsolete and angiography is used very much less, and principally for the evaluation of aneurysms, AVMs, atheroma and other vascular lesions not fully demonstrated by CT. Some tumours may also need angiography for full evaluation. Very detailed studies are required for assessment before interventional techniques such as embolization are undertaken.

Indications and complications

Cerebral angiography carries certain risks and should not be performed without good reason. Where CT scanning is available this would normally be used as the first technique if major neuroradiological imaging is required. Angiography is invasive and should therefore be reserved for cases where CT has failed to provide all the information required. CT does not have sufficient spatial resolution to permit accurate and detailed assessment of aneurysms; extensive angiography is required for these common lesions.

CT will show the number and extent of infarcts but will not provide information about the nature of the cause, such as atheroma, stenosis or embolism, or its location. Angiography may be particularly hazardous in the presence of these latter conditions but may be necessary for a complete diagnosis and particularly where surgical treatment is contemplated.

Arteriovenous malformations are usually readily seen on CT but the diagnosis is not always obvious on the scans. Where doubt exists, and when surgical or radiosurgical treatment is contemplated, then detailed angiography is required to confirm the diagnosis and delineate those blood vessels involved in the lesion.

Venous disorders are uncommon, and are often difficult to diagnose clinically and on CT. Isotope studies may provide further confirmatory evidence, but angiography is usually required to provide a definitive diagnosis. A delayed film series is needed to show the cortical and deep veins to best advantage and to demonstrate venous occlusions and thrombosis.

Prior to CT, angiography was the principal technique used in the diagnosis of brain tumours. CT quickly proved invaluable in this application and the need for angiography dropped sharply. Nowadays the use of angiography in tumours is mostly limited to special applications such as demonstrating the blood supply to meningiomas, defining dural invasion in gliomas, and in differentiating infarcts and low-grade astrocytoma in cases where doubt remains after CT or MRI scans. Certain unusual tumours and those near the base may require angiography for a complete assessment and to exclude other pathology.

Ischaemia and infarction in younger patients may be due to arterial disease other than atheroma, such as arteritis or arteriopathy. Arteriography is often required if these diagnoses need to be confirmed.

Angiography can be hazardous in patients with a previous allergic reaction to contrast media or a history of asthma, hay fever or other allergies. In such circumstances it should only be undertaken after careful assessment of the likely benefits and risks. However, it is generally accepted that intra-arterial injections carry a lesser risk than intravenous in this regard. The amount of contrast medium should be limited to that absolutely necessary to acquire the information needed. The modern low osmolar or non-ionic contrast media should be used wherever possible.

Angiography to diagnose atheroma carries a small but definite risk of embolism and infarction. It is inadvisable, therefore, to undertake angiography in these patients unless the results are likely to materially alter the patient's management. In such cases intravenous digital subtraction angiography may be the safest technique for initial assessment.

Patients who have recently suffered an SAH often have varying degrees of spasm of intracranial vessels. This can be made worse by arteriography and may lead to infarction, or just a general deterioration in the patient's condition. This can be partly overcome by performing angiography immediately or by postponing it until 10 days after the haemorrhage when spasm will usually have diminished. Furthermore, if a significant degree of spasm is seen on angiography, then it is probably wise to restrict the examination to that necessary to acquire essential information.

Apart from those hazards referred to above, arteriography carries other risks associated with the procedure itself. These include haemorrhage or occlusion at the puncture site in the femoral artery. Clots from the catheter, or detached portions of atheroma, may find their way into the vessels of the lower limb or abdomen producing embolic effects. The guide wire may become damaged and fragment, or itself perforate the aorta or other vessels. The catheter may cause subintimal injection of contrast medium in the arterial wall. Fortunately, in experienced hands these complications are unusual and modern arteriography is extremely safe.

When an arteriogram is planned the patient must be properly informed about the procedure and possible risks. A consent form should be signed, and the

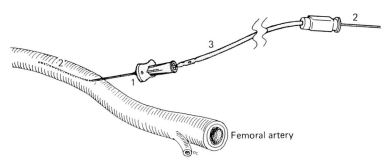

Femoral artery

Figure 51 The femoral artery is punctured with a needle (1); a flexible guide wire (2) is passed through the puncture hole and the needle removed. A catheter (3) is passed over the guide wire into the artery and the guide wire is then removed

patient's groins shaved. General anaesthesia is not usually necessary unless the patient is unable to cooperate, but some form of premedication is desirable. We use an intramuscular injection of Omnopon 10 mg and oral barbiturate 100 mg. A general anaesthetic with controlled hyperventilation will allow fine control of circulation time. Where angiography is unavoidable in a patient with a history of allergy, then antihistamine or steroid cover may be necessary. Following the procedure, monitoring of the patient for changes in neurological status, condition of the puncture site and circulation in the leg, is desirable for 8–12 hours. Complete bed-rest is usually enforced for this period.

Technique

Direct puncture techniques may occasionally be required but will not be described here. Catheter cerebral angiography is usually accomplished via the femoral route. The femoral artery is punctured in the groin with a Seldinger or similar needle. A guide wire is followed with a catheter of at least 100 cm length (*see Figure 51*). Arch injections require a 6 or 7 French calibre catheter of pig-tail or other arch injection type. Selective carotid or vertebral arteriography requires specially shaped catheters (usually 5 French) of which the Mani pattern is the most popular. Other shapes such as Sidewinder, Headhunter etc. may be useful.

For arch studies the tip of the catheter should be placed halfway between the aortic valve and the brachiocephalic trunk. A series of six films is usually sufficient to visualize all the important vessels. A flow-rated pump is desirable for arch injections. A flow rate of 14–16 ml per second and a total volume of 50 ml are sufficient. The patient is usually turned 35°–45° oblique to avoid overlapping of vessels as they arise from the arch. Turning the patient to the left displays the origin of the right common carotid artery and right subclavian artery to best advantage. Turning the patient to the right displays the origin of the left common carotid artery and left subclavian best. Photographic subtraction is essential for a complete

assessment of the vessels, especially those overlying bone. The anatomical features are shown in *Figure 52*.

Selective catheter studies of carotid or vertebral vessels can be obtained with a film series of 1 per second for 6–8 seconds. A more rapid series at 2 per second for the arterial phase and later films at 1 per second will provide more complete visualization of arterial, capillary and venous phases. This is particularly helpful for rapidly shunting lesions such as AVMs and certain tumours. The catheter tip should be placed 2–3 cm above the carotid bifurcation for selective internal carotid injection or about the level of C4/5 in the larger of the two vertebral arteries for vertebral injections. In older patients consideration has to be given to the risk of crossing the bifurcation and if in doubt a common carotid injection should be made. For the intracranial circulation AP and lateral films are the minimum required. Oblique or other projections may also be helpful. Magnification views provide further information but must be done as a routine if they are to be of consistent quality. Doses of contrast medium vary from 6 to 12 ml of around 300 mg iodine per ml depending on the size of the vessel. Hand injections usually provide good visualization but pump injections can be obtained if handled with care (side holes at the catheter tip are then essential to reduce the risk of subintimal injection).

The anatomical features are shown in *Figures 53–59* and some basic angiographic pathology in *Figures 60–63*. Selective studies of the external carotid arteries may occasionally be required. The anatomy of the external carotid artery and its branches are shown in *Figure 53*. The illustrations of angiograms throughout the book have been subjected to photographic subtraction or reversed to provide clearer images and a relatively consistent appearance. The position of right and left are the same as on skull films.

Contrast media have improved greatly in recent years and are safer and more comfortable than ever before. All these studies can be obtained using Iohexol, Iopamidol or Ioxaglate. For arch studies many patients, especially the larger ones, require a higher density medium, e.g. Cardio–Conray.

Angiographic anatomy

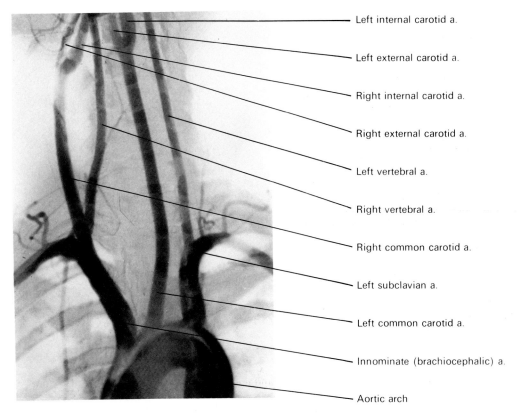

Left internal carotid a.

Left external carotid a.

Right internal carotid a.

Right external carotid a.

Left vertebral a.

Right vertebral a.

Right common carotid a.

Left subclavian a.

Left common carotid a.

Innominate (brachiocephalic) a.

Aortic arch

Figure 52 Aortic arch (oblique)

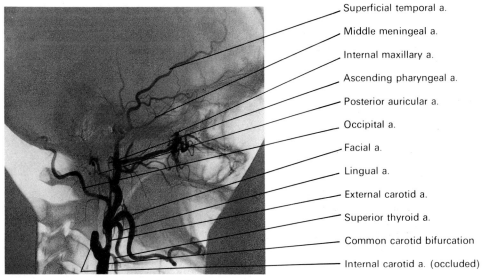

Superficial temporal a.

Middle meningeal a.

Internal maxillary a.

Ascending pharyngeal a.

Posterior auricular a.

Occipital a.

Facial a.

Lingual a.

External carotid a.

Superior thyroid a.

Common carotid bifurcation

Internal carotid a. (occluded)

Figure 53 External carotid artery (lateral)

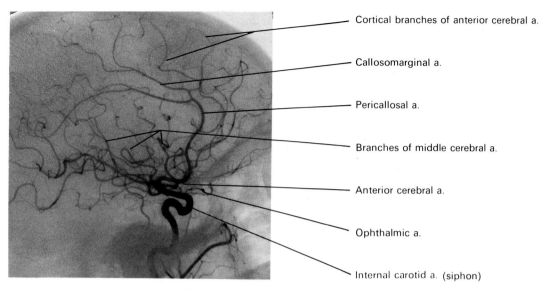

Cortical branches of anterior cerebral a.

Callosomarginal a.

Pericallosal a.

Branches of middle cerebral a.

Anterior cerebral a.

Ophthalmic a.

Internal carotid a. (siphon)

Figure 54 Internal carotid artery (lateral)

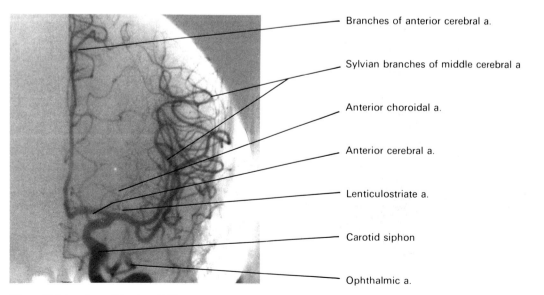

Branches of anterior cerebral a.

Sylvian branches of middle cerebral a

Anterior choroidal a.

Anterior cerebral a.

Lenticulostriate a.

Carotid siphon

Ophthalmic a.

Figure 55 Internal carotid artery (AP)

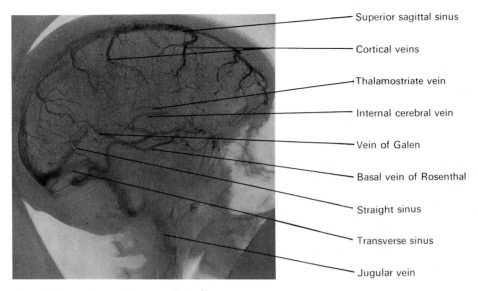

Figure 56 Internal carotid—venous (lateral)

- Superior sagittal sinus
- Cortical veins
- Thalamostriate vein
- Internal cerebral vein
- Vein of Galen
- Basal vein of Rosenthal
- Straight sinus
- Transverse sinus
- Jugular vein

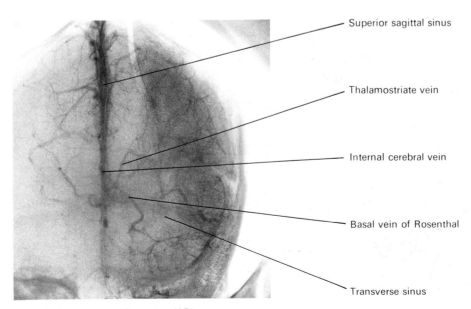

Figure 57 Internal carotid—venous (AP)

- Superior sagittal sinus
- Thalamostriate vein
- Internal cerebral vein
- Basal vein of Rosenthal
- Transverse sinus

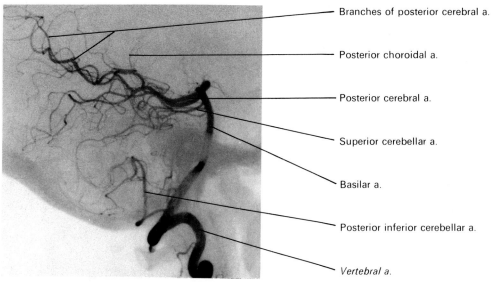

Branches of posterior cerebral a.

Posterior choroidal a.

Posterior cerebral a.

Superior cerebellar a.

Basilar a.

Posterior inferior cerebellar a.

Vertebral a.

Figure 58 Vertebral artery (lateral)

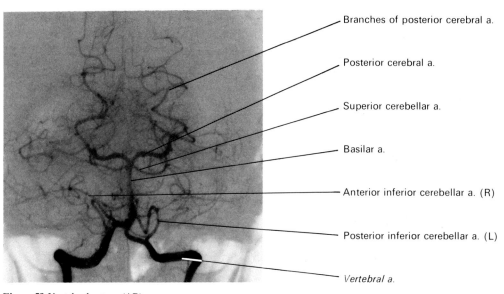

Branches of posterior cerebral a.

Posterior cerebral a.

Superior cerebellar a.

Basilar a.

Anterior inferior cerebellar a. (R)

Posterior inferior cerebellar a. (L)

Vertebral a.

Figure 59 Vertebral artery (AP)

Basic angiographic pathology

Changes on carotid and vertebral arteriography provide considerable information about the vascular structures within the brain and also direct and indirect information about other tissues. Much of this information is discussed in the various sections of Part II. In the pages that follow, some of the basic pathological processes that are demonstrated by angiography are discussed. These include vascular occlusion and arterial disease, vascular shunts, midline shift, vessel displacement and tumour circulation. Aneurysms are discussed in the case presentations.

Diseases of the arteries are very common and the commonest, atheroma, is inevitable with increasing age. This produces narrowing or occlusion of the vessels, and small emboli of atheroma or clots may leave the affected areas and cause occlusion in more distal cerebral vessels. These processes produce transient ischaemic attacks, or complete infarction. The commonest site for atheroma is at the bifurcation of the common carotid in the neck, but all of the arteries shown in the preceding section may be involved.

Under normal circumstances the circulation time from arterial to venous phases on an arteriogram is about 3–5 seconds. Very rapid shunting of blood from arteries directly into veins is seen in a number of situations; the arteries and the veins are then seen at the same time, i.e., on the same film. Such venous shunting is particularly obvious in arteriovenous malformations. Shunting is also seen in blood vessel tumours such as angiomas, in vascular gliomas and in some meningiomas.

The intracranial vessels follow fairly well-established anatomical patterns. A variety of intracranial pathologies cause them to be displaced from their normal position. This displacement provides valuable information about the location of the lesion but, by itself, not much help about the nature of the pathology unless other signs are present.

Many intracranial tumours have increased vascular supply and this feature may aid in their localization and differentiation. This increased supply may be manifested on angiography by tumour vessels, tumour blush or early venous filling. Tumour vessels are additional vessels running to, and within the tumour. They usually show variation in calibre due to encasement by tumour and show no particular arrangement. Tumour blush is a fairly uniform increased density in all, or part of the tumour. Low-grade tumours do not usually show significant tumour circulation (apart from angiomatous masses).

Angiographic pathology

Figure 60 shows an arch aortogram of a patient with multiple areas of narrowing and occlusion of major vessels (arrows). Both internal carotids are occluded. Narrowing is present in the left vertebral artery just above its origin and at the origin of the left common carotid from the arch. This patient has severe generalized arterial disease and has recently suffered a major stroke.

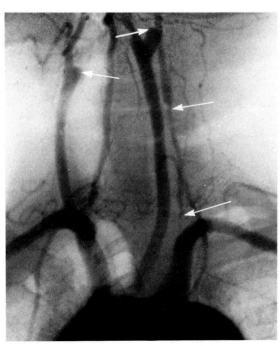

Figure 60

Figure 61 shows a lateral film from an angiograph series. This arterial phase film shows a large circumscribed knot of dilated vessels in the territory of the middle cerebral artery. Two larger vessels lead away from the lesion on the other side from the arteries. These are large draining veins from this arteriovenous malformation. The arteries and veins are simultaneously filled on the same film indicating the rapidity of the shunt.

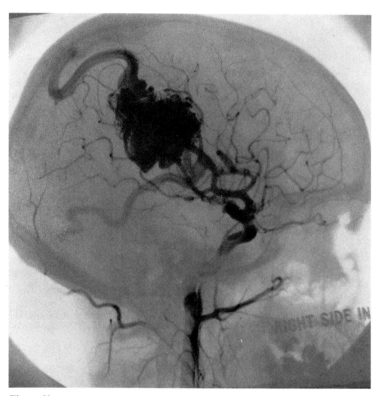

Figure 61

Figure 62 is an AP projection arterial phase film from another patient. The anterior cerebral vessels are displaced from their normal midline position towards the right side. The left middle cerebral vessels are displaced upwards and stretched over a mass lesion below them. A zone of abnormal vessels and 'staining' is present in this area due to a tumour.

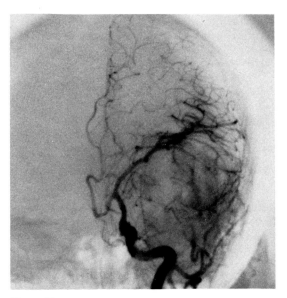

Figure 62

Figure 63 is a lateral film in the venous phase of a patient with a tumour in the upper hemisphere. The pattern of the cortical veins is deficient in the frontoparietal area and some of the adjacent veins are stretched along the anterior aspect of the mass which also shows a faint tumour blush.

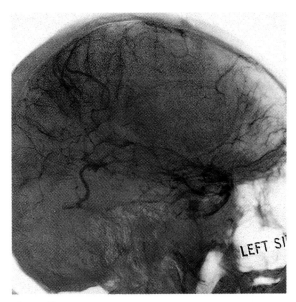

Figure 63

Computerized axial tomography (CT)

CT is now recognized as one of the greatest advances in diagnosis since the discovery of X-rays. Since its development in 1972, CT quickly became established as the foremost, and often the only technique required to diagnose brain pathology. Air studies consequently became obsolete and angiography was required much less often. Furthermore, CT provides us with anatomical and pathological detail not possible through other techniques, short of craniotomy; in many instances further invasive diagnostic procedures are not required.

Image generation and display

CT brain scan images are produced by computerized reconstruction of a slice of head tissues which has been analysed by a moving X-ray beam. The patient lies comfortably on a couch with his head in the aperture of the gantry (*Figure 64*). This contains the X-ray tube and detectors which generate digital information from each slice. This digital information is then processed by the computer to produce the images. Depending on the machine, each slice takes from 10 to 60 seconds to examine, and a full routine examination about 20–60 minutes. The procedure is quite painless, but some patients may require a further set of 'enhanced' scans after an intravenous injection of an iodinated contrast medium (similar to that used in intravenous urography). Introduction of air or contrast medium into the subarachnoid spaces or ventricles may also be used to provide further information in certain special situations. Most modern scanners can also perform body scans.

Each image represents a slice of brain tissue and these are presented in sequence from the base of the brain upwards. A slice is usually 5–10 mm thick and normally touches its companion cuts on either side so that reviewing a sequence of slices in order enables one to build up a mental picture of the whole brain. The standard position of the slices and their visual sequence are shown (*Figure 65*). Many modern machines are capable of scanning (or recalculating the data) into other planes, e.g., sagittal or coronal.

The image and its densities

The CT brain scan is capable of displaying all the range of densities between air and bone, indeed this range is present on most images in clinical use. Air is shown as black and bone as white, with all the intervening densities as varying shades of grey. The values of grey can be adjusted by varying the settings (known as window width and level) on the imaging system, but for most purposes and throughout this book the settings used are constant to avoid confusion.

The densities encountered on the majority of scans are shown in *Figure 66* (their approximate numerical values in Hounsfield units are given).

The CT images reproduced here are mostly from two machines, the EMI 1010 Head Scanner and an up-to-date GE 8800 Body Scanner. Most of the conditions shown can be readily diagnosed on quite basic CT scanners. All CT scans in this book are

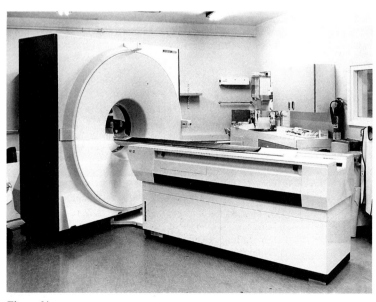

Figure 64

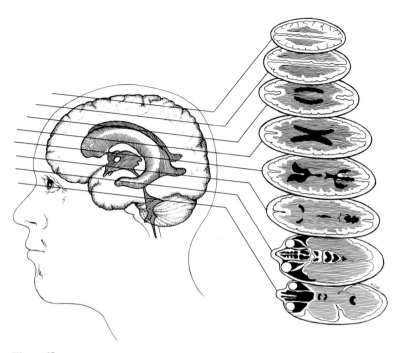

Figure 65

−1000	Air	}	difficult
−100	Fat	}	to distinguish
0	Water		
0–10	CSF		
12–18	Brain oedema		
22–32	White matter		
35–45	Grey matter		
55–75	Haemorrhage		
80–200	Calcification	}	difficult to
200–1000	Bone	}	distinguish

Figure 66

displayed with the patient's left side on the left of the image and the face at the top. Images showing '[+C]' represent a contrast-enhanced scan.

Scan supervision and interpretation

Special preparations are not required for most patients having brain scans. Patients should however be kept fasting for 4 hours prior to the scan as some will require an injection of iodinated contrast medium (contrast enhancement) and this may produce some nausea. All patients should be reassured and the procedure explained to them; restless or unco-operative patients will probably require sedation.

The indications for CT brain scanning are numerous and include: suspected head injury, tumour, stroke, infarct, intracranial infection, hydrocephalus, etc. Scanning of epileptic patients and those with dementia will reveal underlying pathology in some cases. The extent to which such problems can be evaluated by CT is governed by available resources.

The standard unenhanced scan should produce 8–10 consecutive slices of 8–10 mm thickness from the lower posterior fossa to the vertex. These images should be assessed for any lesion, and to see if any area of brain has been omitted. Most focal lesions need to be enhanced, as do most patients with suspected metastases, orbit, pituitary or posterior fossa lesions. The purpose of enhancement is to improve the pick-up rate of lesions and to provide further information about the lesions that are visible on the plain scan. Contrast enhancement usually involves a bolus intravenous injection of a suitable iodinated contrast medium. In some departments this is given by infusion. After this, the scan series is repeated. The contrast medium renders many vascular structures visible and other lesions also show an increased density in specific patterns. This is due to the presence of multiple small abnormal vessels and/or a breakdown in the blood–brain barrier allowing the dense contrast material to enter the lesion. The plain scan effects of lesions include dilatation of one or more ventricles (hydrocephalus), compression, or displacement of those ventricles and midline structures (mass effect). The lesions themselves may be the same density as brain (isodense), or of higher or lower density than brain. The position of a lesion, its density, effects on surrounding structures and pattern of enhancement, together with clinical details, all help to provide facts on which a probable diagnosis can be based. These aspects are covered throughout the case discussions.

It must be clearly understood that contrast enhancement, like intravenous urography, carries a small but significant risk and should only be given where clear indications for its use exist.

It is important to realize that brain disorders, like most other things in nature, do not always conform to the 'rules' and the diagnosis may not be 'cast-iron' from the scans. Follow-up scans are very helpful in clarifying the situation, as the progress of a lesion over a period of time is usually an index of its character.

Anatomy

The anatomical features shown on any particular slice depend on a number of factors, including the thickness and position of the slice, the angulation of the head during scanning and the quality of the scanner. The illustrations on the following pages show fairly typical slices of 10-mm thickness, consecutively arranged from the skull base to the vertex. The head angulation used was standard at about 15 degrees to the canthomeatal line. The images were generated on a state of the art scanner (GE 8800) and represent quality close to the maximum possible with current technology. Only the important structures are identified, as detailed anatomical analysis is beyond the scope of this book. Variation of the head angulation will include different combinations of structures on individual slices, other than those shown here. Thinner slices help to reduce artefacts and give finer detail. These are particularly useful in the posterior fossa, sella turcica and orbit. Coronal and sagittal CT images, either directly produced or from reformatting of axial scan data, are not included in this book. A short selection of some common normal variants and artefacts follows the anatomical images. Anatomy images in *Figures* 77 and 78 show some normal anatomical features visible on contrast-enhanced scans.

Basic CT scan pathology

The range of pathological processes revealed on CT scans is vast and much of this will be covered in Part II. In the section that follows the anatomy images, some of the fundamental pathological changes are demonstrated, e.g., hydrocephalus, mass effects, low-density and high-density lesions, and enhancement. These may be present individually, in combination with each other, or with more subtle signs.

CT anatomy

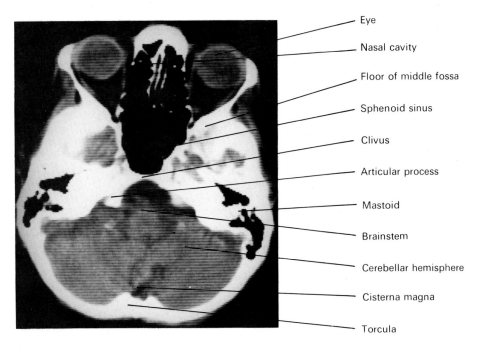

Eye

Nasal cavity

Floor of middle fossa

Sphenoid sinus

Clivus

Articular process

Mastoid

Brainstem

Cerebellar hemisphere

Cisterna magna

Torcula

Figure 67

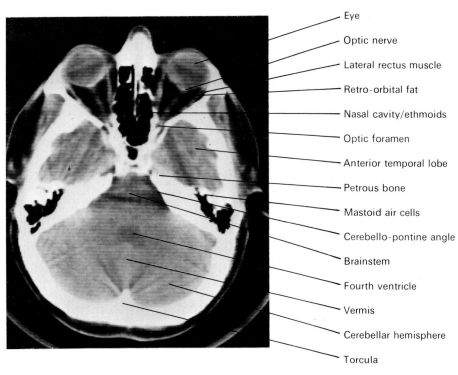

Eye

Optic nerve

Lateral rectus muscle

Retro-orbital fat

Nasal cavity/ethmoids

Optic foramen

Anterior temporal lobe

Petrous bone

Mastoid air cells

Cerebello-pontine angle

Brainstem

Fourth ventricle

Vermis

Cerebellar hemisphere

Torcula

Figure 68

40

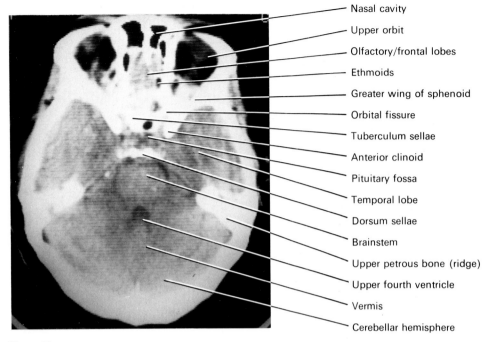

Nasal cavity

Upper orbit

Olfactory/frontal lobes

Ethmoids

Greater wing of sphenoid

Orbital fissure

Tuberculum sellae

Anterior clinoid

Pituitary fossa

Temporal lobe

Dorsum sellae

Brainstem

Upper petrous bone (ridge)

Upper fourth ventricle

Vermis

Cerebellar hemisphere

Figure 69

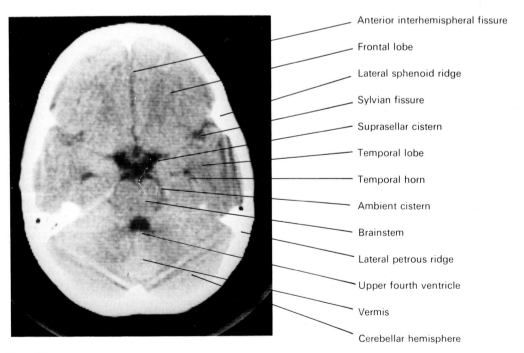

Anterior interhemispheral fissure

Frontal lobe

Lateral sphenoid ridge

Sylvian fissure

Suprasellar cistern

Temporal lobe

Temporal horn

Ambient cistern

Brainstem

Lateral petrous ridge

Upper fourth ventricle

Vermis

Cerebellar hemisphere

Figure 70

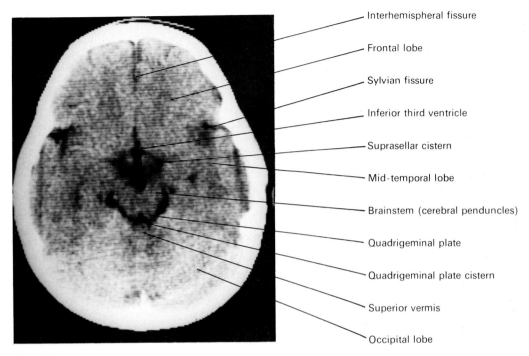

Interhemispheral fissure

Frontal lobe

Sylvian fissure

Inferior third ventricle

Suprasellar cistern

Mid-temporal lobe

Brainstem (cerebral penduncles)

Quadrigeminal plate

Quadrigeminal plate cistern

Superior vermis

Occipital lobe

Figure 71

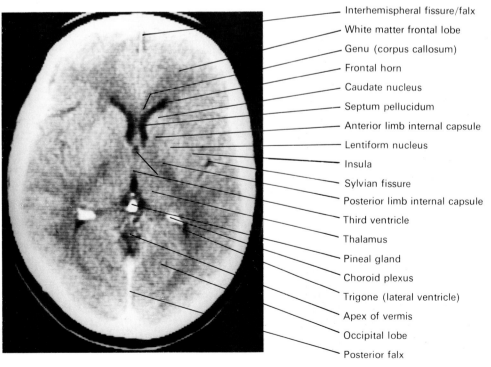

Interhemispheral fissure/falx

White matter frontal lobe

Genu (corpus callosum)

Frontal horn

Caudate nucleus

Septum pellucidum

Anterior limb internal capsule

Lentiform nucleus

Insula

Sylvian fissure

Posterior limb internal capsule

Third ventricle

Thalamus

Pineal gland

Choroid plexus

Trigone (lateral ventricle)

Apex of vermis

Occipital lobe

Posterior falx

Figure 72

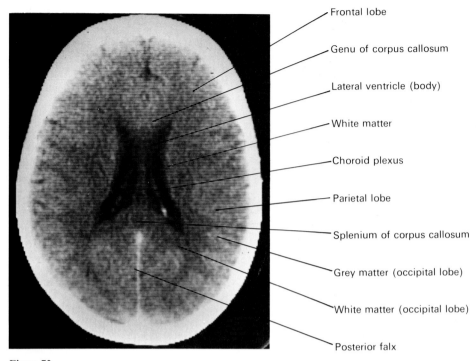

Frontal lobe

Genu of corpus callosum

Lateral ventricle (body)

White matter

Choroid plexus

Parietal lobe

Splenium of corpus callosum

Grey matter (occipital lobe)

White matter (occipital lobe)

Posterior falx

Figure 73

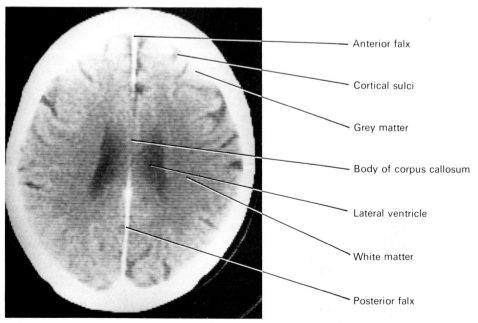

Anterior falx

Cortical sulci

Grey matter

Body of corpus callosum

Lateral ventricle

White matter

Posterior falx

Figure 74

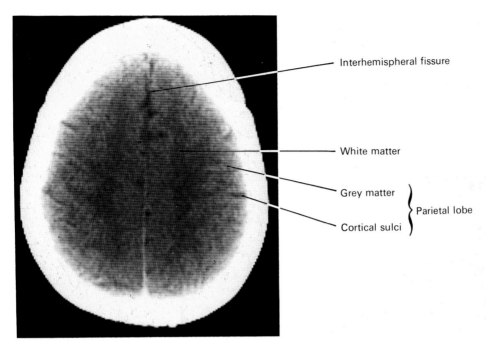

Interhemispheral fissure

White matter

Grey matter

Cortical sulci

} Parietal lobe

Figure 75

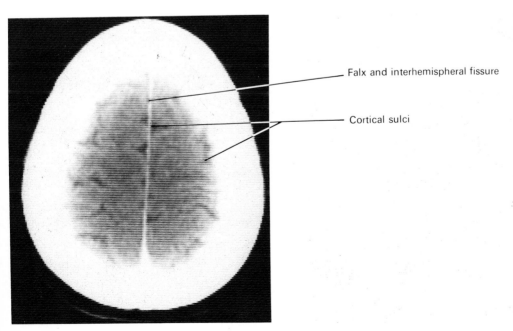

Falx and interhemispheral fissure

Cortical sulci

Figure 76

44

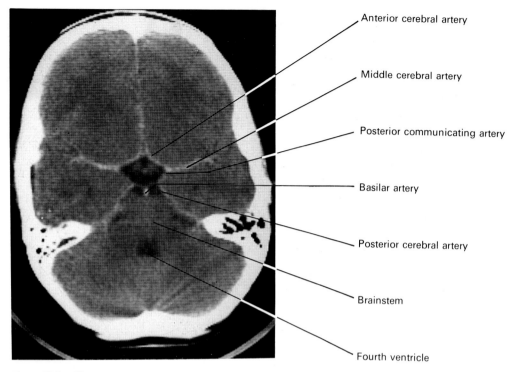

Anterior cerebral artery

Middle cerebral artery

Posterior communicating artery

Basilar artery

Posterior cerebral artery

Brainstem

Fourth ventricle

Figure 77 [+C]

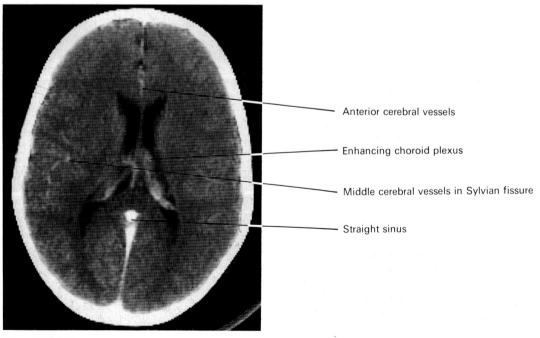

Anterior cerebral vessels

Enhancing choroid plexus

Middle cerebral vessels in Sylvian fissure

Straight sinus

Figure 78 [+C)

CT artefacts and variants

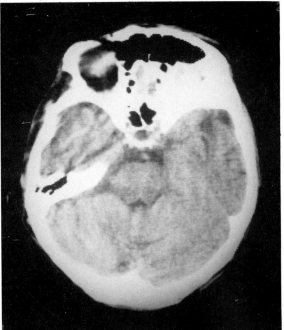

Figure 79

Figure 79 shows asymmetry of the petrous bones. The one on the right is not visible. This is due to the patient being incorrectly placed in the scanner, with his head tilted to one side. This is confirmed by the asymmetry of the orbits. The main importance of this artefact is that it makes cerebral structures look odd at higher levels.

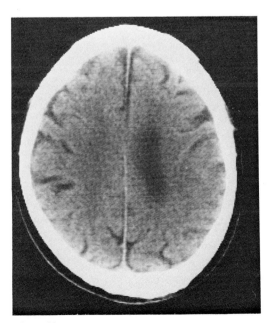

Figure 80

Figure 80 shows the same patient as in *Figure 79* with a scan through the upper ventricles showing how the asymmetrical placing of the head makes the brain look as though there is a mass effect in the left hemisphere. This pitfall can be avoided by routinely examining lower slices for evidence of asymmetry of the bony outlines.

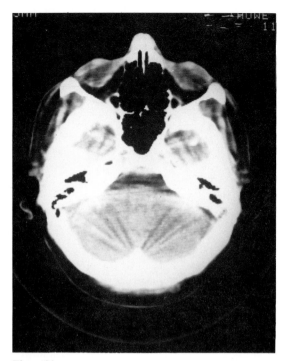

Figure 81

Because of the high proportion of bone to brain in these low slices (*Figure 81*) many images of the posterior fossa and middle fossa are impaired by streak artefacts. The horizontal black band between the petrous bones is common and is called a Hounsfield band. The radiating streaks from the torcular are also commonly seen. Both middle fossae also show diagonal band artefacts from the petrous bones.

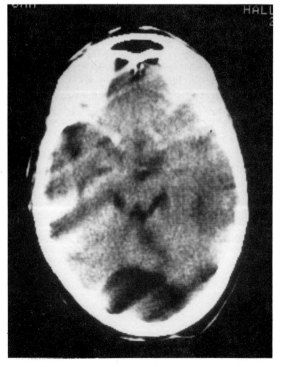

Figure 82

The diagonal streaks across the whole head in *Figure 82* are due to a restless patient moving his head while the scan is being taken. This problem can usually be overcome by reassurance or adequate head fixation. Sedation may be required. This patient also has a congenitally large cisterna magna. This is of no consequence and should not be confused with a Dandy–Walker syndrome (*see* Case 98).

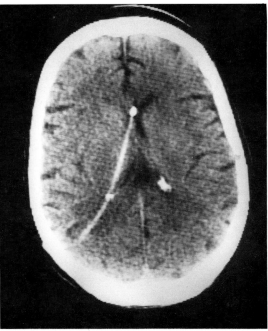

Figure 83

The scan in *Figure 83* shows a dense line running into the left lateral ventricle with a larger dense end in the frontal horn. This is a shunt tube inserted for the relief of hydrocephalus (successful!). It emerges through a burr hole in the parietal bone (not visible at this level). The appearance of these tubes is variable, but the position and density of this one are fairly typical.

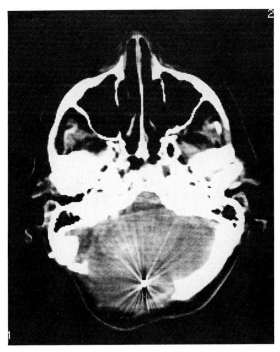

Figure 84

A large bone defect is noted in the left side of the posterior fossa in *Figure 84*. This is due to previous surgery (craniotomy). A very dense artefact close to this and associated with radiating streaks is due to a piece of metal. Such densities may be the result of surgical clips or foreign bodies such as bullets. The contrast medium Myodil (Ethiodan) used in myelography often leaves small densities scattered in the basal cisterns.

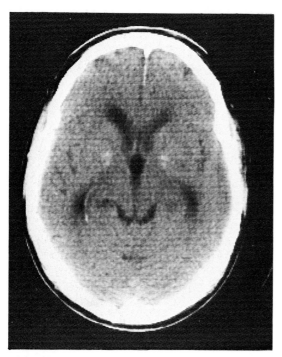

Figure 85

Figure 85 shows symmetrical calcification in the basal nuclei. This is a normal finding in many people and is associated with increasing age. More florid examples, especially if associated with calcification in nuclei in the cerebellum, suggest a disorder of calcium metabolism (hypoparathyroidism).

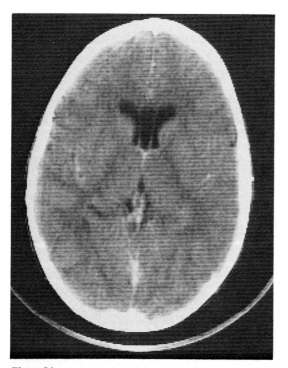

Figure 86

The thin septum separating the frontal horns of the ventricles is called the septum pellucidum. The normal appearance can be seen in *Figure 72*. *Figure 86* shows a common variant of the septum where the normal membrane is in two parts with an intervening cyst. This is known as 'cavum septum pellucidum' or simply a 'cyst of the septum pellucidum'. A variant, also normal, may be seen at the posterior end of the third ventricle—the 'cavum septum vergae'.

CT pathology—mass effect/hydrocephalus

Many cases of intracranial pathology produce their symptoms and cause CT changes by virtue of their mass effect. The cranial cavity is a rigid box and processes which take up space within it cause other structures to be displaced away from their normal position, and/or compressed. This often affects their function and that of other adjacent structures. *Figure 87* shows structures which are normally situated in the midline displaced to the left side (septum pellucidum). The right lateral ventricle is compressed and displaced to the left side of the midline. There is, therefore, a 'space-occupying' process in the right side of the head producing this mass effect. This lesion can be seen as a low density area outside the hemisphere due to a chronic subdural haematoma.

Ventricular dilatation (hydrocephalus) is clearly demonstrated on CT. The lateral, third and fourth ventricles are clearly shown and although formal measurements are possible, their size can usually be assessed by experience. Most cases are the result of obstruction to normal CSF flow and the pattern of dilatation may help to indicate the site of the problem, e.g., large lateral and third ventricles and a small fourth ventricle often indicate an aqueduct obstruction (*see Figure 88*). Unilateral dilatation of one lateral ventricle may be seen in obstruction of a foramen of Munro, but is often due to distortion of that structure by midline shift.

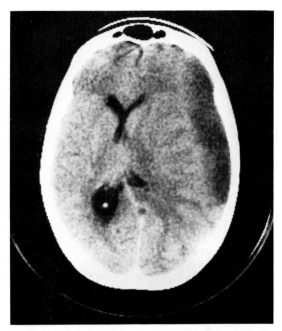

Figure 87

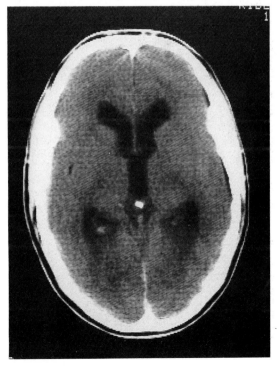

Figure 88

CT pathology—low density lesions

The most common response of brain tissue to the presence of some disease process is for it to show an area, or areas of decreased density. This is partly due to brain oedema around the lesion, or the lesion itself being of lower density than brain. The standard display of CT images represents these lesions as being darker than surrounding brain. It is important, however, not to confuse these with structures, such as CSF spaces and white matter, which are normally of low density.

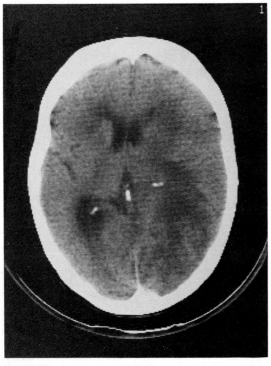

Figure 89

Figure 89 shows such a lesion in the right occipital lobe, where patchy low density is present. The calcified choroid plexus and trigone are displaced forwards indicating an associated mass effect. The enhanced appearance of this lesion is shown in *Figure 93*.

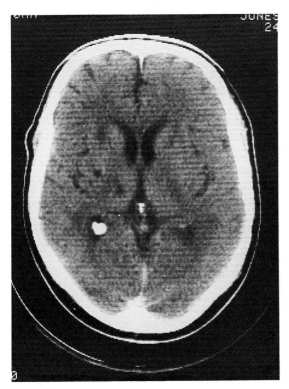

Figure 90

Figure 90 shows further low-density lesions. These are situated in the left thalamus and internal capsule, and are clearly defined with no associated mass effect. This appearance and location is very suggestive of small infarcts. There are few other conditions that can account for such an appearance.

CT pathology—high density lesions

A variety of densities that have higher Hounsfield numbers than brain tissue may be encountered. The commonest of these are: (i) densities marginally greater than brain, e.g., meningioma, (ii) freshly extravasated blood as in haematoma and (iii) calcification. *Figure 91* shows a well-defined vague area of increased density in the lower right frontal lobe just above the skull base. There is a zone of low density (oedema) surrounding this lesion. This is the marginally raised density of a meningioma. The enhanced appearance is shown in *Figure 94*. (Note the dilated temporal horn on the left.)

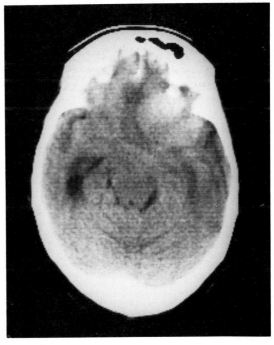

Figure 91

Figure 92 shows an area of strikingly high density in the left thalamus. This patient had a sudden onset of headache and right hemiparesis and this is the appearance of an acute intracerebral haemorrhage. This condition is further discussed in Case 23. Density as high as this is difficult to distinguish from calcification but a measurement of Hounsfield numbers within the area will help to differentiate these two conditions (*see Figure 66*).

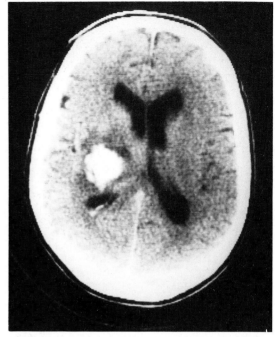

Figure 92

CT pathology—contrast enhancement

Following the administration of an iodinated contrast medium, many brain lesions show areas of increased density when compared to the unenhanced scan. This density is the result of two processes present in many brain lesions: (i) increased perfusion by blood vessels supplying the lesion or the affected adjacent brain, and (ii) breakdown of the normal blood–brain barrier, thus allowing contrast medium to leak into and opacify the affected tissue. The pattern of enhancement seen in brain pathology is often quite characteristic, and when assessed in conjunction with the other data on the scans can provide vital clues about the diagnosis.

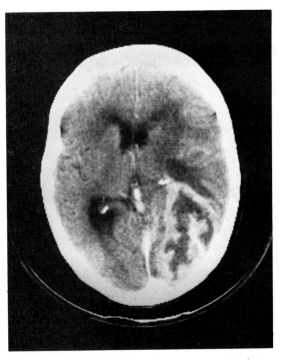

Figure 93 [+C]

Figure 93 shows an enhanced scan on the patient in *Figure 89*. This previously low-density area has now opacified irregularly, both around its margins and centrally. The appearances are practically diagnostic of malignant glioma and other possible causes for the plain-scan appearance such as abscess or focal oedema can be excluded.

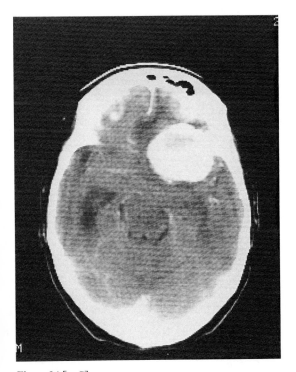

Figure 94 [+C]

Figure 94 shows an enhanced scan on the patient in *Figure 91*. The well-circumscribed area of slightly increased density has enhanced uniformly and markedly: further conclusive characteristics of a meningioma.

Intrathecally enhanced CT

Occasionally conventional CT scanning does not provide all the information required about certain lesions. This is particularly true of small lesions in the basal cisterns. It may then be helpful to introduce an intrathecal contrast agent, either iodinated contrast medium or air. This will provide further and more detailed anatomical and pathological information. These media are introduced by lumbar or cervical puncture and run up into the basal cisterns by tilting the patient head down for a few minutes on a myelography table.

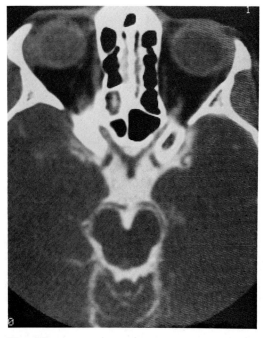

Figure 95

Figure 95 shows a scan from such an examination. The CSF which is normally low density on a scan now appears white (high density). Structures lying within the subarachnoid spaces are now more clearly visible. The optic chiasm and optic nerves can clearly be seen as a 'V-shaped' filling defect just above the pituitary fossa. Just lateral to this area the carotid siphons can also be seen on each side. Posteriorly the brainstem with the individual cerebral peduncles is outlined by the opacified CSF. The posterior cerebral arteries can be seen running around the cerebral peduncles.

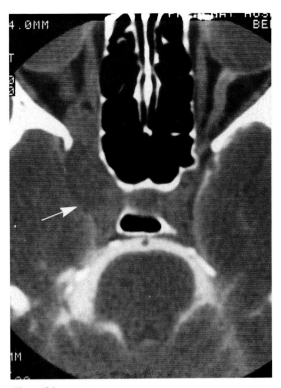

Figure 96

Figure 96 is a further example of this technique. The opacified CSF outlines the upper pons and the basilar artery can be seen as a small filling defect in the contrast medium. On the right side of the pituitary fossa the CSF outlines the lateral margin of the cavernous sinus. On the left this area is enlarged and distorted (arrow) by a cavernous sinus lesion which also extends anteriorly into the orbit. This was a tumour of nerve sheath (Schwannoma).

This technique can also be used to study variations in CSF flow in cases of hydrocephalus (*see* Case 90).

Magnetic resonance imaging (MRI)

MRI is the latest in a long and imaginative series of technological advances which have been put to work in the service of medical diagnosis. Its success represents a brilliant triumph for an exemplary blending of modern engineering and dedicated scientific and clinical research. Although the images produced by this technique are superficially similar to CT, the physical and biological principles involved are very different. The information it provides is quite unlike that previously available and some understanding of this imaging system is necessary.

MRI is based on the physical phenomenon called nuclear magnetic resonance (NMR). This was described by Bloch and Purcell working independently in the USA in 1946. They discovered that certain atomic nuclei, when placed in a uniform magnetic field and subjected to a brief pulse of radiofrequency, emit a pulse of radiofrequency (RF) in response. This 'resonance' can be measured and contains information about the stimulated nuclei. This exciting development was quickly applied to the analysis of chemical samples (spectroscopy) and has been extensively used in this field ever since. In the early seventies, Damadian, Lauterbur and other researchers described methods of using these physical concepts to produce images representing body tissues in a manner similar to that of CT. The ultimate goal of MRI may be the blending of spectroscopy and imaging in a single technique.

The patient is placed inside a powerful magnet and a series of radiofrequency pulses are initiated. The body tissues contain atomic nuclei which behave as 'small magnets' and respond at resonance to produce an RF signal which is detected and stored. By varying the magnetic field and the RF pulse all the resultant data can be processed to produce images of the body tissues. Since the hydrogen nucleus (proton) produces the strongest signal, and is found in all body tissues, this is the one currently used for imaging. It is possible to detect other nuclei, such as phosphorus, in the body, but imaging from these nuclei is still only in the research phase.

It is important for the reader to note that the science of MRI is highly complex and evolving rapidly. Changes in the understanding and application of this technique are occurring almost daily. The descriptions which follow are necessarily over-simplified and, furthermore, many of the concepts will inevitably be superseded as new research emerges. This is particularly likely in the case of pulse sequences and systems for data acquisition.

Basic physical and biological principles

Many atomic nuclei can be considered to act as spinning magnetic dipoles (*Figure 97A*). This model is an over-simplification, but will suffice for an understanding of the basic principles of NMR.

When the tissue under examination is placed within the powerful magnetic field the latter causes some of the nuclei to align the axis of their spins along the force field (*Figure 97B*). A dynamic equilibrium exists with the nuclei precessing about their axes at a resonant frequency known as the Larmor frequency. This Larmor frequency is directly proportional to the applied magnetic field and specific to the nucleus under examination. The magnetization vector is then briefly rotated (usually through 90° or 180°) by application of an RF pulse tuned to the Larmor frequency (*Figure 97C*) and will subsequently return to its original equilibrium direction. The tissue acquires energy during this pulse with the spinning nuclei now

aligned in the new field (excitation) and precessing in phase with each other. This energy is released as the magnetization vector returns to its original alignment ('relaxation') (*Figure 97D*). The emission of energy is in the form of a brief faint pulse of RF. This signal is detected and stored; its characteristics reflect the quantity and state of the atoms in the tissue. (The 'exciting' RF pulse and the point in time at which the resonant signal is measured can be infinitely varied and is known as the *pulse sequence*.)

In the case of MRI the atom under study is hydrogen which has a single proton for its nucleus. This is the most abundant proton in human tissue and therefore provides the best opportunity for a useful detectable signal. Two-thirds of the body hydrogen is contained in water molecules. The remainder is present in fats and proteins. Body water is therefore the principal source of signal and the overall amount of water in a tissue is reflected in an MRI parameter known as *proton density*. Some of this water is bound to the surface of protein molecules. This binding restricts the ability of these protons to relax following excitation and this phenomenon leads to two other resonance characteristics which may be represented on MR images, namely *T1 and T2 relaxation times*.

The *T1 relaxation time* is dependent on the time

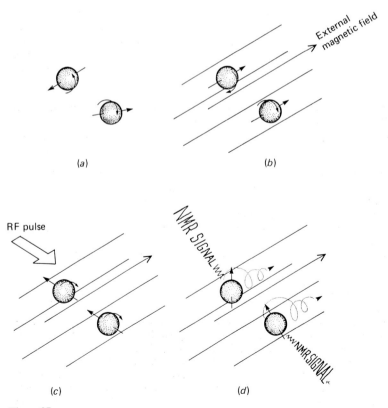

Figure 97

taken for magnetization to return to equilibrium and reflects the loss of energy by the nuclei to their local environment. Broadly speaking the greater the proportion of free water present, the longer the T1 relaxation time will be. Conversely, when the proportion of bound water is highest then T1 will be shorter. This has an important practical application, as many different pathologies cause increased free water in the tissues and hence a prolonged T1.

The *T2 relaxation time* is dependent on nuclear spins going out of phase with those surrounding them. This parameter is particularly sensitive for the detection of disease processes. As in the case of T1 an increase of free water causes a prolongation of T2 relaxation time.

A further parameter which is finding increasing clinical applications is *flow effects*. When moving blood is magnetized it has moved on before the resonant signal is received and leaves a signal void at the appropriate site on the image. This makes it possible to identify vessels intracranially and elsewhere, and quantitative flow measurements are also possible.

These MRI parameters—proton density, T1, T2, and flow effects—are currently the most important components in the MR image. The images can be manipulated to give particular emphasis to one or more of these parameters by an appropriate choice of *pulse sequence*.

Other useful imaging parameters are being identified such as 'susceptibility' and 'chemical shift'. These are beyond the scope of this book.

Technical details

MRI requires a powerful magnetic field of uniform strength. This may be provided by a permanent magnet but most clinical systems use either a conventional electromagnet (resistive) or super-conducting magnet (cryogenic). The former are cheaper but are effectively limited to field strengths around 0.15 tesla (0.15 T). Super-conducting systems are super-cooled using liquid helium and nitrogen. These can provide field strengths in the range 0.25–2 T or more. Although good images can be obtained using field strengths of 0.15 T, it appears that the highest quality of images requires at least 0.5 T (1 T = 10 000 gauss). The earth's magnetic field is of the order of 0.00005 T.

The patient lies within the bore of the main magnet (*Figure 98*). The RF required to alter the direction of the magnetization vector during each pulse is transmitted through a saddle-shaped copper coil near the patient. This coil may also be used to receive the resonant signal, but for accurate local studies (e.g., spine) surface coils are used. This emitted signal contains a variety of data relating to protons in many different locations. Consequently, some system has to be present to allow the scanner to locate the source of

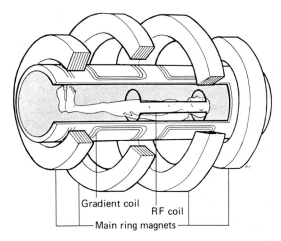

Gradient coil   RF coil
Main ring magnets

Figure 98

the data within the body, thereby permitting build-up of images based on the MRI signal and spatial information. This is achieved using additional magnet coils (gradient coils) which cause the main magnetic field to be slightly varied along the three coordinates (gradients) (*Figure 98*). By matching the frequency (MHz) of the RF pulse to those magnetic gradients the computer defines longitudinal spatial data enabling selection of a specific slice of tissue for study. Data acquired in the other planes permit reconstruction of an image map of the varying MR signals within that slice. These are called *spatial and phase encoding*. The repetitive switching of the gradients during the scanning process accounts for the audible noise within the scanner.

The time required to acquire sufficient signal to produce a useful image is quite long and a series of slices would take proportionally longer. During each pulse cycle there are periods when nothing is happening while the instrument waits for tissues to equilibrate again before the next pulse is applied. This makes it possible for adjacent slices to be excited without interfering with the slice that is returning to equilibrium. This is known as simultaneous or *multiple-slice acquisition* and most modern scanners use variants of this technique to acquire multiple adjacent slices simultaneously. This greatly reduces overall examination time.

Pulse sequences

MR images are dependent on the parameters mentioned in the preceding section, namely, proton density, T1 relaxation, T2 relaxation and flow effects. The extent to which these are reflected in the image depends on the pulse sequence used. Many types of sequence have been described and no doubt many more will be developed, some of which may replace those currently most popular. The three sequences described below represent the basic formats used in current clinical practice. It is also possible to image for more than one sequence at a time.

The pulse sequence is made up of one or more excitation RF pulses followed after a specified interval by a period during which the resonant signal is received; after a further interval the whole process is repeated. The various time intervals are critical and are measured in milliseconds. They are: TR (repetition time), time for one complete cycle; TE (time to echo), time from initial RF pulse to resonant signal; TI (time to inversion), time from initial RF pulse to second inverting pulse (*see* inversion recovery sequence). These may be represented as shown in *Figure 99* in a hypothetical (but quite useless) pulse sequence.

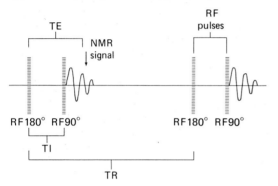

Figure 99

Saturation recovery (SR). In this sequence an RF pulse aligns the magnetization vector to 90°. The resonant signal is then measured and the whole process repeated. This may be illustrated as shown in *Figure 100*.

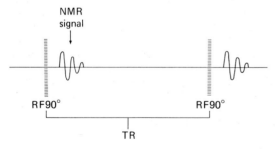

Figure 100

Whichever pulse sequence is used, the signal is in the form of a diminishing oscillation and is called free induction decay (FID). When TR is long, then the signal only contains proton density information. For a short TR the protons are not fully equilibrated before the next RF 90° pulse arrives and the signal contains some T1 information, but is rather weak. This sequence is little used in clinical practice since the other sequences provide sufficient proton density information.

Inversion recovery (IR). In this sequence two RF pulses are applied: the first swings the magnetization vector through 180° and after a short interval ('time to inversion' or TI) the vector is inverted by a 90° pulse. Following this the resonant signal is measured and then after a further interval the process is repeated. This may be represented as illustrated in *Figure 101*.

The second pulse catches many protons partially relaxed and the resultant signal contains much useful T1 data as well as proton density. This sequence is time-consuming (and increasingly so with higher field strengths), but because white/grey matter differentiation is dependent on T1 discrimination it provides excellent anatomical delineation. A typical sequence might be TR = 1400, TI = 400: this would be written 1400/400.

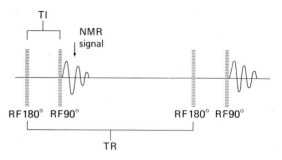

Figure 101

Spin-echo (SE). In this sequence an initial RF pulse swings the magnetization vector through 90°. This is followed by a 180° pulse. This combination results in an initial signal after the 90° pulse which is ignored and the 180° pulse then causes the nuclei to rephase their spins. The 180° pulse is timed to occur at the midpoint between the 90° RF pulse and the second signal. This may be illustrated as in *Figure 102*.

The resultant signal contains a variable amount of T1 and T2 information. The amount of T1 data in the resultant image can be altered by varying the length of TR (shorter TR and TE = more T1). The amount of T2 data in the image is dependent on TE, there being more T2 when TR and TE are long. The sequence has

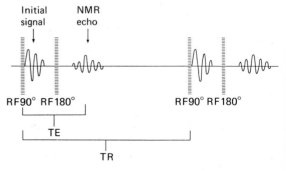

Figure 102

many variants and some centres use it exclusively to provide T1 or T2 'weighted' images as it can be performed more quickly than IR sequences. T2-weighted images are the most suitable for demonstrating diseased tissues. A typical T1-weighted sequence might be $TR = 500$, $TE = 30$: this would be written 500/30. A typical T2-weighted sequence would be 2000/80. Although images can be weighted towards relaxation characteristics (T1 and T2), the image will always be a function of proton density and the resulting contrast between tissues may also be affected by other paramerers such as flow.

Special considerations

Certain practical problems attend the use of powerful magnetic fields and RF pulses in MRI. Problems on site include interference by and on the field, due to extraneous ferromagnetic materials. Vehicles, steel girders, etc. may cause problems in achieving a uniform magnetic field and the siting of the magnet is critical. Conversely, the magnetic field creates problems within a certain radius depending on the field strength. Computer discs and tapes, credit cards, watches, oscilloscopes, etc. may be damaged by the field. Movable ferromagnetic objects such as scissors, keys, screwdrivers and anaesthetic equipment may move towards the magnet bore at dangerous speeds and must be excluded from the area. Extraneous RF sources may also affect the instrument, and extensive shielding may be needed. So far as the patient is concerned, the magnet field may alter pacemaker rhythms, dislodge cochlear implants and cause intracranial ferromagnetic aneurysm clips to undergo torsion; such patients should be excluded from the vicinity of the magnet. Other surgical clips do not appear to present any hazard. Metallic objects such as hairpins, jewellery or dentures may cause local degradation of the image, or become detached and turn into projectiles.

The patient lies within the bore of the magnet. This space is like a tunnel and may give rise to claustrophobia. The sound from gradient switching may also add to the apprehension. A full explanation and reassurance are usually all that is required, but some patients may need sedation. Observation and monitoring of the patient may be difficult and anaesthesia creates special problems. Data acquisition is considerably slower than with CT and examinations involving several pulse sequences and anatomical planes may take an hour or more.

Indications

As the technology, clinical understanding and application of MRI evolve, so the extent of its contribution to diagnosis widens. In the years to come it may well become the prime technique for the diagnosis of brain disorders. While the number of scanners remains limited however, and examination times are long, its use may have to be limited to situations where it has distinct advantages over CT. At present the applications include: the study of white matter disease, especially multiple sclerosis; lesions at the base including pituitary masses; lesions in the posterior fossa; abnormalities of the cranio-cervical junction. Examples of these applications are included in the case studies.

Anatomy and pathology on MRI

To a large extent the anatomy seen on MRI is very similar to that on CT, but different tissues show varying signal intensities on different pulse sequences. A structure showing high signal on IR sequences may show low signal on SE and so on. Direct coronal and sagittal imaging is also readily achieved and the anatomical relationships in these planes need to be considered in addition.

As described earlier, an inversion recovery sequence produces images which contain both proton density and T1 information. The overall signal intensity of all sequences is proportional to proton density. Bone has a low proton density and shows a low signal on all sequences although marrow has a high fat content which shows a high signal on most sequences. Although many disease processes cause changes in proton density, this is usually a less important feature of the image than the changes in T1 and T2 which are more pronounced.

CSF has a very long T1 and appears black on inversion recovery sequences. Grey matter has a moderately long T1 and also appears quite dark. White matter has a short T1 and appears white (high-signal) (see Figure 107). Most pathological lesions have long T1 and appear dark on IR sequences. The exception to this is early haemorrhage and lipid, both of which have short T1 (high-signal) and appear white.

CSF also has a very long T2. It, and lipid, have high signal (white) on T2-weighted sequences. CSF can be made to appear dark by using a short TE. The signal from CSF may also be changed due to flow effects. Most lesions also show high signal. The T2 and proton density values for grey and white matter are quite similar and these tissues are not as readily separated on T2-weighted sequences.

Contrast agents

Contrast enhancement, in a similar fashion to that of CT, can be achieved using paramagnetic agents. These are not imaged directly in the tissues, but by their effect on the local relaxation times. These agents are still the subject of much research. The most promising appears to be a chelate of gadolinium, i.e., Gd.DTPA. This produces signal changes due to increased perfusion and blood–brain barrier penetration, and has been shown to help in the delineation of tumours from their surrounding oedema. The future role of contrast agents in clinical practice has yet to be established.

MRI anatomy—axial plane

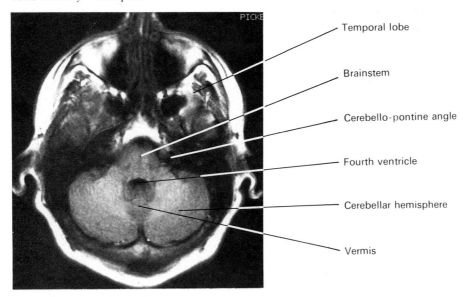

Figure 103 Posterior fossa (IR)

Temporal lobe

Brainstem

Cerebello-pontine angle

Fourth ventricle

Cerebellar hemisphere

Vermis

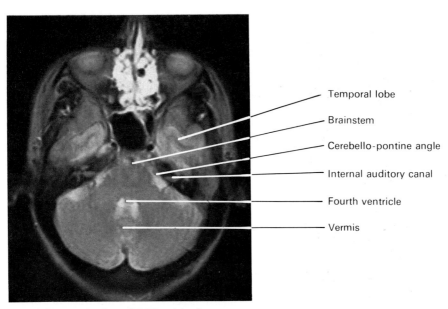

Figure 104 Posterior fossa (SE T2-weighted)

Temporal lobe

Brainstem

Cerebello-pontine angle

Internal auditory canal

Fourth ventricle

Vermis

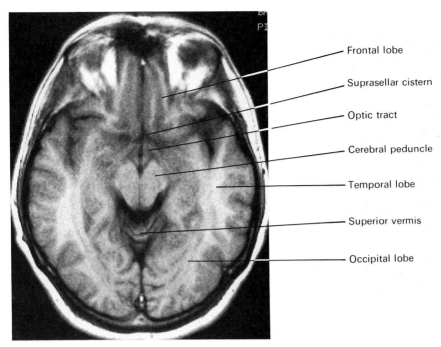

Frontal lobe

Suprasellar cistern

Optic tract

Cerebral peduncle

Temporal lobe

Superior vermis

Occipital lobe

Figure 105 Suprasellar (IR)

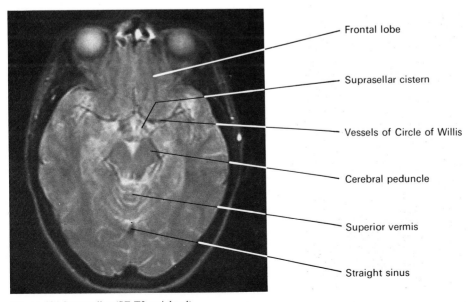

Frontal lobe

Suprasellar cistern

Vessels of Circle of Willis

Cerebral peduncle

Superior vermis

Straight sinus

Figure 106 Suprasellar (SE T2-weighted)

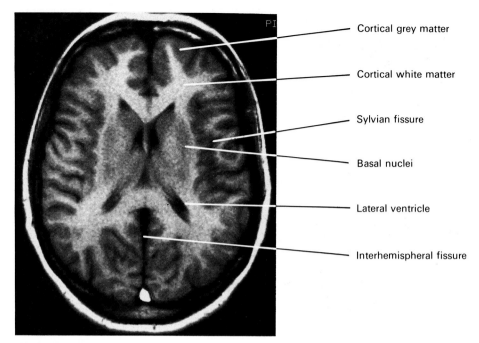

Figure 107 Cerebral hemispheres (IR)

Cortical grey matter

Cortical white matter

Sylvian fissure

Basal nuclei

Lateral ventricle

Interhemispheral fissure

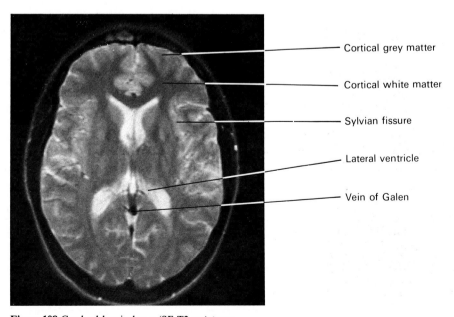

Figure 108 Cerebral hemispheres (SE T2-weighted)

Cortical grey matter

Cortical white matter

Sylvian fissure

Lateral ventricle

Vein of Galen

MRI anatomy—coronal plane

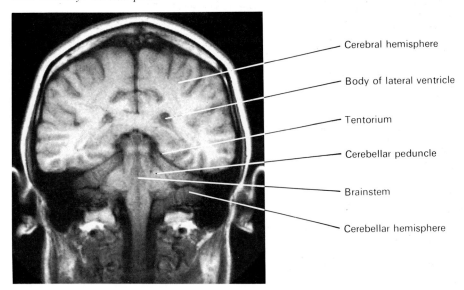

Cerebral hemisphere

Body of lateral ventricle

Tentorium

Cerebellar peduncle

Brainstem

Cerebellar hemisphere

Figure 109 Brainstem (IR)

MRI anatomy—sagittal plane

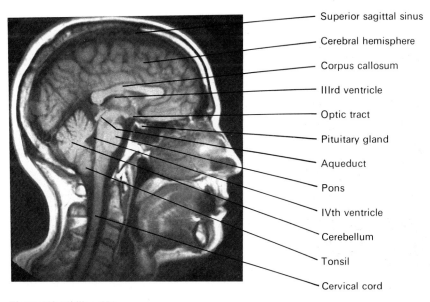

Superior sagittal sinus

Cerebral hemisphere

Corpus callosum

IIIrd ventricle

Optic tract

Pituitary gland

Aqueduct

Pons

IVth ventricle

Cerebellum

Tonsil

Cervical cord

Figure 110 Midline (IR)

Part II—The cases

Subacute or recurrent headache

General considerations

Headache is one of the commonest symptoms in clinical medicine, whether the patient consults a general practitioner or specialist. The diagnostic possibilities are many, but most cases can be diagnosed by taking a careful history and examination. In only a few cases is further investigation necessary. A useful generalization is 'the shorter the history of headache, the more likely is the possibility of a serious cause'. Apart from this factor other important features include the site, quality, duration, frequency, mode of onset, associated symptoms and aggravating or relieving factors. For the purpose of this book, headaches of 5 days' duration or less are considered to be 'acute'.

Headache is produced in a variety of ways. The principal mechanisms are:

1. *Vascular*. These include migraine, temporal arteritis, fever: vasoconstriction and/or vaso-dilatation stimulate nerve endings and cause release of pain-producing substances into the scalp.

2. *Muscular*. These are due to muscular spasm in the cervical muscles causing pain to radiate over the head.

3. *Inflammatory*. Inflammation of the meninges by meningitis or SAH; usually produce severe headache. This is mostly from the pain-sensitive meninges along the base of the brain.

4. *Traction*. Distortion of intracranial anatomy by hydrocephalus, or mass effects due to focal oedema, haemorrhage or tumour all produce headache.

5. *Disease of nearby structures*. These include pain referred along cranial nerves from lesions in the eyes, ears, sinuses, teeth, bone, etc.

Headaches that are recurrent in type are almost invariably benign. Causes include migraine, tension headaches, chronic sinusitis, dental or oral problems and post-traumatic headache. Intermittent obstruction of the CSF pathways due to an intraventricular tumour acting as a ball-valve is an important exception. Consequently, any recurrent headache where attacks are encountered only in certain positions of the head is worthy of further investigation. Migraine is the commonest cause of recurrent headache and the pain is usually unilateral, associated with nausea, vomiting and often preceded by an aura. Only in cases with associated focal neurological disturbances such as dysphasia or weakness should diagnostic imaging be required to exclude other diagnoses or migrainous complications such as cerebral ischaemia. Tension headaches, probably the result of muscular spasm, are characterized by a long history and often recur every day with a pressure-band sensation. An anxiety state or depression is often present. Chronic sinusitis and other congestive mucosal disorders are common causes of chronic headache: confirmatory evidence can be found in an allergic rhinitis-type history and visible changes in the nasal passages. A variety of dental problems including mild displacement of the temporomandibular joints from ill-fitting dentures may produce headache, although the oral source of these is usually obvious on close questioning.

Post-traumatic headache is common and may follow what is often only a trivial injury. The mechanism here is poorly understood, but the history of the injury is usually readily forthcoming. It is important however to remember the possibility of a structural cause such as a chronic subdural haematoma or post-traumatic hydrocephalus. The presence of appropriate neurological signs will suggest that definitive diagnostic imaging techniques should be employed, namely CT.

Subacute headache is rather more serious and raises

the possibility of a range of sinister intracranial pathologies. Any prolonged headache that is progressive in severity, or occurs in a person not normally subject to such symptoms, is a cause for concern. Furthermore, if there is evidence of drowsiness, raised intracranial pressure or any focal neurological change, then an intracranial lesion is likely. In these circumstances, plain skull films may be helpful in revealing evidence of raised intracranial pressure, midline shift, intracranial calcification, etc. CT scanning will be the principal method of diagnosis, although isotope scanning may reveal evidence of many of the gross lesions. MRI scanning or angiography may be helpful in selected cases. The more important of these lesions are listed below.

Temporal arteritis is an important differential diagnosis of headache in patients over the age of 55. Most cases are fairly obvious with systemic upset and tenderness over the affected vessel. However, some cases are more indolent and the true diagnosis may not be immediately apparent. Diagnostic imaging is not normally indicated in this condition but cerebral infarction may occur and be the presenting feature. The syndrome of benign intracranial hypertension is not well understood and is usually encountered in women, but also in children of both sexes. A history of headache is associated with evidence of papilloedema in the absence of other neurological signs. Imaging may be required to exclude other diagnoses. The

ventricles are normal or small in size. This condition (also known as pseudotumour cerebri) may be due to a number of causes including obesity, sinus thrombosis and certain drugs.

Some of the commoner causes of recurrent or subacute headache with imaging manifestations are listed below. The first 12 are described on the following pages, the remainder are discussed under other clinical presentations.

Malignant glioma
Oligodendroglioma
Meningioma
Subdural haematoma
Metastases
Epidermoid/dermoid
Neurofibroma
Arteriovenous malformation
Intracranial granuloma
Hydrocephalus:
   aqueduct stenosis
   pinealoma
   posterior fossa mass
   colloid cyst (Case 18)
   brainstem tumour (Case 78)
Malignant astrocytoma (Case 30)
Pituitary masses (Case 73)
Intracranial cysts (Case 44)
Metastases in skull base (Case 60)

Case 1

Male, aged 47 years.
Eleven-week history of intermittent headache.
Two generalized convulsions during last 2 weeks.
Early papilloedema.

Q: What logic underlies further investigation of this patient?

Q: Images A, B and C were obtained in this case, what are they and what do they show?

Q: What might angiography be expected to have shown in this case had this been available?

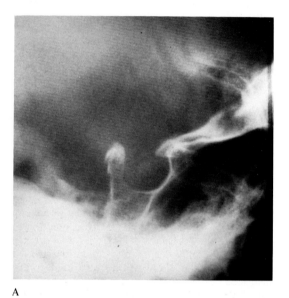

A

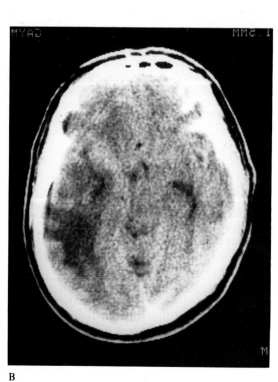

B

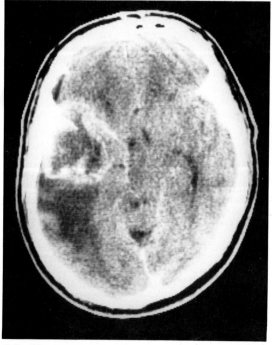

C [+C]

Case 1   Malignant glioma

In this patient the presence of papilloedema suggests optic neuritis (also a cause of headache) or raised intracranial pressure. The latter possibility certainly warrants further studies. The recent onset of fits in an adult is also very disturbing and usually requires further investigation.

Image A is part of a lateral skull film and shows some erosion of the posterior margin of the pituitary fossa (*see Figure 5* for normal appearance). This indicates raised intracranial pressure of several weeks' duration confirming that the finding of papilloedema is indeed very significant. Images B and C are plain and enhanced CT scans respectively, and show an extensive low density area in the left frontotemporal region. This extends medially into the basal nuclei and is producing considerable space-occupying effect resulting in marked shift of midline structures to the right. The contrast-enhanced scan shows an irregular rim of enhancement lying within this area of low density. The diagnosis is that of malignant glioma.

Malignant glioma is the most rapidly growing and invasive of the tumours of glial tissue. As a group these glial tumours are the commonest intracranial neoplasms after metastases and comprise a spectrum of lesions ranging from slow-growing 'benign' astrocytomas through more aggressive 'malignant' astrocytomas to this lesion, also known as 'glioblastoma multiforme'. The history is fairly short, some patients only experiencing symptoms for a few weeks. Weakness, sensory loss, headaches, fits and even psychological disorders may be the presenting features, singly or in combination (*see* Case 94). Progression is rapid, surgical removal is often incomplete and the recurrence rate is high even with radiotherapy. They may occur anywhere in the brain but the most malignant lesions are unusual in the posterior fossa. Less malignant gliomas are described in Cases 30 and 39.

The CT appearances are typified by this case. The margin of the enhancing area is usually irregular in outline and varies in thickness. This appearance should be compared with that of a brain abscess where the enhancement is more ring-like and shows a consistent thickness (*see* Case 17). The tumour provokes a zone of surrounding oedema and the outer margin of the tumour tissue is probably close to the outer edge of the enhancing area. Enhancement is due to a combination of tumour vessels and local leakage of the contrast medium. Deep within the lesion an area of lower density may be seen due to cyst formation or necrosis. Mass effect is almost invariably present. The differential diagnosis includes abscess, solitary metastasis, granuloma or infarction. Metastases rarely get to this size and a primary may already be manifest. Granulomas, although rare, can look very similar to this and are most likely due to tuberculosis. Infarction does not produce this degree of mass effect and follows a distribution pattern appropriate to a vascular territory (*see* Case 22).

Plain films may show evidence of midline (i.e., pineal) shift, calcification within the tumour, or raised intracranial pressure. Isotope studies will show non-specific uptake in the tumour. Arteriography in this more malignant grade of tumour is not normally necessary since the CT appearances are so specific. An angiogram would show midline shift and locally displaced vessels together with tumour circulation. The latter would appear as irregular proliferated vessels and early venous shunting (*see Figure 62*). However, an abscess or metastatic deposit could look similar. It seems likely that MRI will be at least as sensitive and probably more so than CT in detecting such tumours. Delineation of the margin between tumour and oedema may not be possible even with gadolinium enhancement.

Case 2

Female, aged 54 years.
Ten-month history of headache.
Recently several generalized fits.

Q: Images A and B are from a CT scan performed on
    this patient. What do these scans show, and what
    is the relevance of plain film C?

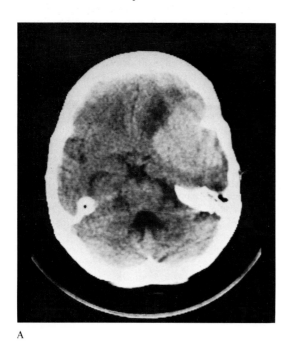

A

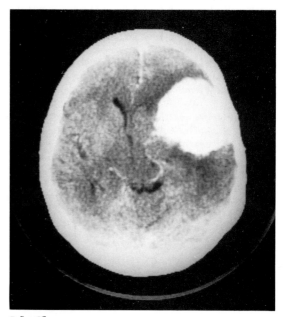

B [+C]

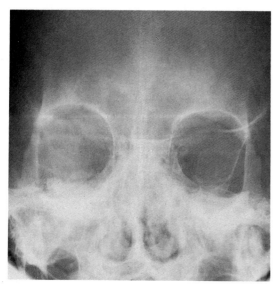

C

Case 2   Meningioma

Although a long history of headache is often an indication that the cause is unlikely to be serious, in this case the recent fits add further concern and detailed investigation is indicated. The plain scan shows a well-defined area of slightly increased density with surrounding oedema in the right frontotemporal area. Its close relationship to the lateral margin of the greater wing of sphenoid should be noted. The enhanced scan shows a fairly uniform increased density throughout the lesion. The appearances are typical of meningioma.

This common benign tumour arises from the meningeal coverings of the brain (diagram E, *see below*). Typical sites at which it may be found include the convexity (A), falx (B), olfactory groove (C), sphenoid ridge (D), tuberculum sella (E), tentorium (F) and cerebello-pontine (CP) angle (G). A mass arising in such a location should always be suspected of being a meningioma. They may also be encountered within the ventricles. Meningioma is a slow-growing tumour and may be present for many years before the diagnosis is made. Headache and a variety of other symptoms may be produced depending on the location of the tumour. An accurate diagnosis is important however, as this lesion is potentially curable following surgical removal.

Most meningiomas are uniform in consistency but may show cyst formation or calcification (visible on plain films). These tumours draw the bulk of their blood supply from meningeal vessels: arteriography will show hypertrophied meningeal arteries and a uniform tumour blush. In cases where doubt exists about the diagnosis on CT, or where surgeons require information about the vascular supply prior to surgery, then arteriography can be very helpful. Image D shows the arteriogram on this patient with a hypertrophied middle meningeal artery (arrow) supplying the vascular tumour. The prominent vascular supply at the tumour's attachment to the meninges often provokes thickening in the underlying bone. This is called enostosis and may be visible on plain films. Image C shows this change in the greater wing of sphenoid on the right, where thickening of the bone has rendered the right orbit more dense than the left. Isotope scans show well-defined uptake. Meningiomas may be difficult to identify on MRI but further work on pulse sequences and gadolinium enhancement should overcome this problem. Other manifestations of meningioma and possible causes of similar CT appearances are discussed in Cases 28 and 72.

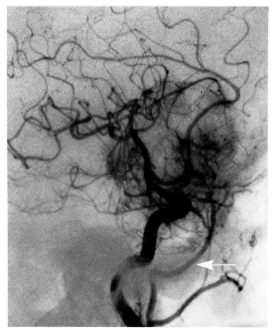

D

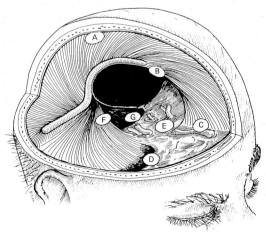

E

Case 3

Female, aged 51 years.
Seven-month history of headache.
Recently mild confusion.

Q: What diagnostic technique is this, and what possible diagnosis does it suggest?
Q: How might you finalize the diagnosis?

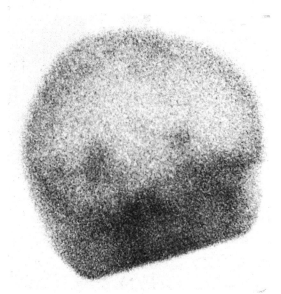

A

Case 3   Metastatic disease

This is a lateral view of an isotope brain scan. Compare this image with a normal brain scan in *Figure 48*. There are a number of areas of increased uptake of isotope. The commonest cause for this appearance is multiple metastases within the brain substance, but other lesions can produce an identical picture. These include multiple abscesses, meningiomas or infarcts. Multiple neuromas can be demonstrated by isotope techniques but do not show this degree of uptake.

The brain is a common site for metastatic deposits. These most frequently arise from primary tumours in the lung or breast, and from malignant melanoma. The majority of these grow in the cerebral substance. They also occur in the meninges (*see* Case 43), and deposits in bones of the skull base may produce headache or local pressure on the cranial contents (*see* case 60). Deposits within the cerebral substance produce a wide variety of clinical syndromes including headache, seizures, dementia, hemiparesis, posterior fossa signs, etc., depending on their location.

Plain films of the chest and skull may reveal valuable confirmatory evidence of a primary, or other secondary tumours. CT scanning is the principal technique used for imaging brain metastases. The characteristic feature is their multiplicity. Most lesions have surrounding oedema and are themselves less dense than brain. Almost all metastatic deposits show definite enhancement and post-contrast scans should always be obtained when this diagnosis is suspected. Following enhancement the lesions may be solid or have a ring-like structure. Consequently, metastatic deposits can look similar to glioma, abscess or infarction, especially when a single lesion is present (*see* Case 41). Biopsy may be necessary for a final diagnosis. A small number of lesions are denser than brain (*see* Case 43). Angiography usually reveals local mass effect with some evidence of tumour circulation.

Images B and C below are from an enhanced CT scan and show ring-like enhancement in two metastatic lesions in the cerebellum. The lesion in image C is in the upper vermis with the enhancing margin of the tentorium forming curved high-density lines around it.

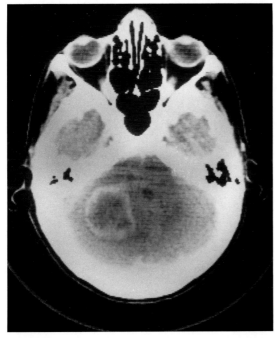

B [+C]

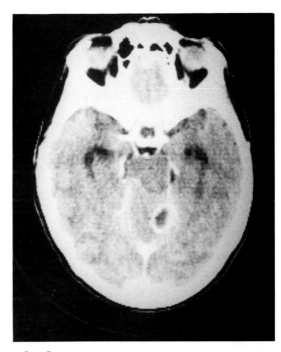

C [+C]

Case 4

Female, aged 22 years.
Headaches for 3 years.
Recently some cranial nerve signs.

Q: What diagnostic technique was used for scans A–
    C, and what do the images show? Can you
    identify the relevant technical parameters?
    (Image D is a CT scan on this patient.)

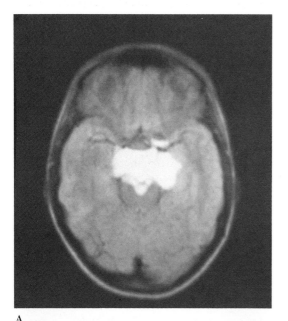

A

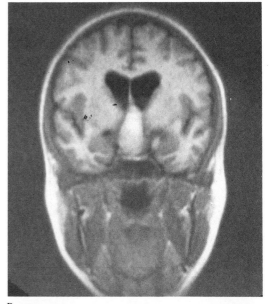

B

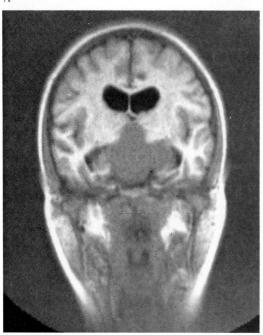

C

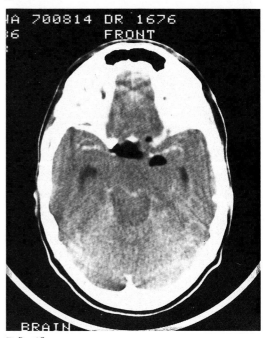

D [+C]

Case 4   Intracranial dermoid

Images A, B and C are from an MRI scan. Image A is an axial scan through the suprasellar area. The pulse sequence is a T2-weighted spin-echo study. This is apparent from the bright signal derived from the cortical grey matter and lower signal from white matter (*see* Part I). This image shows an area of high signal intensity (long T2) in the suprasellar cistern extending laterally on both sides with posterior distortion and compression of the cerebral peduncles. Images B and C are coronal scans from the same examination, but using an inversion recovery sequence (T1-weighted). This sequence can be deduced from the dark cortical grey matter, lighter white matter and black CSF. Image B is more anterior and shows the anterior temporal lobes with dilated ventricles. A high-signal mass (short T1) is present in the region of the third ventricle. Image C is a slice obtained more posteriorly and passes through the temporal horns of the lateral ventricles. An extensive low-signal mass extends between them and up into the posterior third ventricle. This part of the lesion corresponds to the high-signal area on image A and indicates a well-defined but non-specific mass. The high signal (short T1) in the anterior third ventricle on image B is very suggestive of fat. This mixture of solid and fatty components in a midline lesion is highly suggestive of a dermoid tumour.

There is a spectrum of intracranial tumours which are derived from primitive germinal tissues. These are not common, but since they are benign a cure is theoretically possible and their diagnosis is therefore very important. Tumours derived from epidermis contain keratin and are called 'epidermoids' (*see* Case 33). Lesions derived from all skin layers are called 'dermoids' and may contain skin, hair, fat or calcium. This case contains fat and solid elements and so belongs to this group. Dermoids are usually found in the midline but also occur in the vault (*see Figure 28*). Hamartomas contain dermal elements but may also exhibit bone, muscle or abnormal blood vessels. These latter may be difficult to differentiate from dermoids, but dense calcification and areas of enhancement may be evident on a CT scan.

Because of the history of cranial nerve deficit in this case, it would have been quite appropriate to have obtained MR first. However, because of the availability of resources, a CT scan was obtained initially. A representative axial slice is shown in image D. The areas of very low density are characteristic of fat. The most interesting feature here is how much more extensive the lesion appears on the MRI scans. This is particularly evident in the posterior part of the lesion which is poorly delineated on CT, but is accurately defined on MRI. The coronal images are particularly helpful in this respect.

Case 5

Female, aged 28 years.
History of headaches for $2\frac{1}{2}$ years.
Mild papilloedema.

Q: Plain film A was obtained on this patient. What
   abnormality is shown, and how does this relate to
   image B?

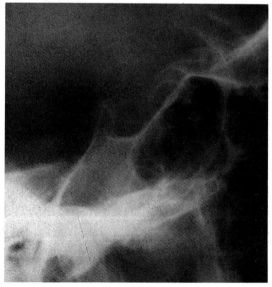

A

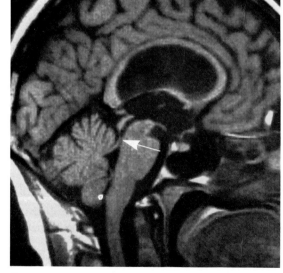

B

Case 5   Aqueduct stenosis

Image A is from a lateral skull film. The pituitary fossa has been deformed into a 'J' shape. This is the result of pressure on the anterior superior wall of the fossa in the region of the tuberculum sellae. The pressure is produced by downward bulging of a dilated third ventricle and this sign indicates the presence of hydrocephalus. A similar deformity, with which this should not be confused, is seen with pressure from a glioma of the optic chiasm ('omega' sella, Case 59). This appearance is highly suggestive of aqueduct stenosis.

Aqueduct stenosis is a major cause of hydrocephalus. The aqueduct is stenosed (probably as a result of a developmental defect) and a hydrocephalus develops affecting the third and lateral ventricles. The fourth ventricle is not involved and like the rest of the posterior fossa contents may be rather small. The condition may present at any age from early childhood to late adult life. The hydrocephalus can be tolerated for years without symptoms until some other illness or trauma upsets the delicate balance. In the very young the presentation will be that of increasing head circumference and perhaps retarded development. Older patients usually present with headache and may show signs of raised intracranial pressure. CT scanning provides good delineation of the ventricular changes with dilated third and lateral ventricles, and a normal fourth. These features are shown on the CT scan from this patient in images C and D below. The major differential diagnosis of the CT appearance is aqueduct obstruction by tumour. Contrast enhancement should be given and any anatomical distortion noted. Many surgeons require delineation of the stricture with contrast medium within the ventricles, but MRI may make this procedure unnecessary. Image B is a T1-weighted sagittal MRI scan on this patient. The aqueduct is visualized above the fourth ventricle and the narrowed segment is clearly demonstrated (arrow).

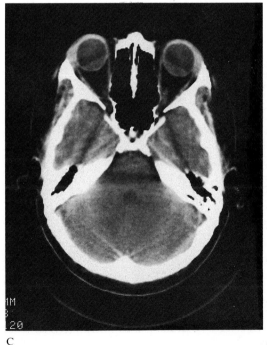

C

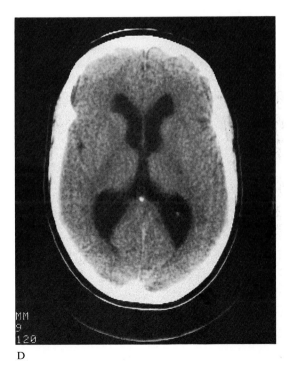

D

Case 6

Female, aged 37 years.
Headaches of 3 months' duration.
More recently nausea and vertigo.

Q: Because of the history of vertigo a CT scan was
    obtained. Images A and B are from that study.
    What do they show?
Q: Can you make a definitive diagnosis from these
    images?

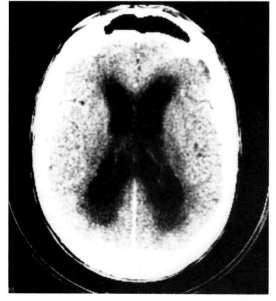

A

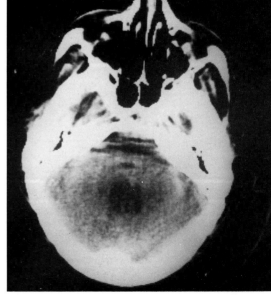

B

Case 6   Hydrocephalus due to posterior fossa tumour (astrocytoma)

Image A shows dilated lateral ventricles. There is no associated sulcal widening to suggest atrophy and the zone of interstitial oedema ('flare') around the ventricles suggests that this is an obstructive hydrocephalus (*see* Case 90). Image B shows an ill-defined low-density area in the expected site of the fourth ventricle. A cursory study of these images might deceive one into thinking this was a case of communicating hydrocephalus (*see* Case 63) since all four ventricles appear dilated. However, the low-density area in the posterior fossa is not the ventricle, as this structure can be seen as a dark slit compressed and displaced forwards by this lesion. The diagnosis of hydrocephalus is incomplete as the cause may be a lesion in the posterior fossa. Contrast enhancement is therefore indicated. Image C is from the post-enhancement study on this patient and a ring of irregular increased density can now be seen within the area of low density. Ring-like enhancement can suggest an abscess but the history is really too long for this. A granuloma such as tuberculosis is a possibility although rare outside endemic areas. The appearances are more likely to be those of a tumour. In this age-group an enhancing low-density tumour in the midline

of the posterior fossa is most likely to be a cerebellar astrocytoma. While this lesion's low density helps to differentiate it from other midline posterior fossa tumours such as medulloblastoma (Case 79) or ependymoma (Case 80), it is most likely to be confused with haemangioblastoma (Case 86) or cerebellar infarction (Case 81). A metastatic deposit is also a possibility.

Cerebellar astrocytoma usually runs a more benign course than its counterparts above the tentorium and is the commonest primary cerebellar tumour in children and young adults. The lesion is commonly cystic and may be found in the vermis (midline) or cerebellar hemispheres. Ring-like enhancement is the usual pattern and hydrocephalus is commonly present. Plain films may show evidence of raised intracranial pressure. Isotope studies will demonstrate non-specific uptake; angiography would be expected to show displacement of posterior fossa vessels and possibly some tumour circulation. MRI will probably prove to be the most useful diagnostic technique due to its superior demonstration of posterior fossa structures.

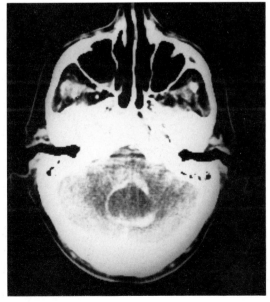

C [+C]

Case 7

Male, aged 63 years.
Three-week history of headache.
More recently, bouts of confusion.

Q: A definitive imaging technique was performed
and representative images are shown in A and B.
What firm diagnosis can you make?

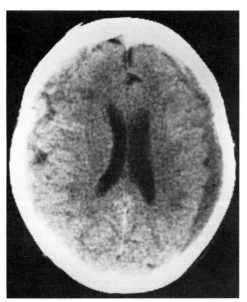

A

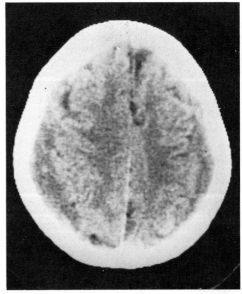

B

Case 7   Chronic subdural haematoma

These images are part of an unenhanced CT scan. Image A shows a shallow low-density collection lying outside and over the surface of the right hemisphere. The ventricles are displaced to this side, inappropriate to this mass effect. This could be due to atrophy on the right (for which there is no evidence, e.g., sulcal widening or focal ventricular dilatation) or a mass effect on the left. Image B was taken at a higher level and shows the cause of this shift as there is now evidence of another collection over the upper left hemisphere. These two collections are of different densities and are the result of chronic subdural haematomas.

This condition is a consequence of head injury (often only minor) which produces a small acute haematoma in the subdural space by a shearing tear of the bridging veins. Mostly such lesions present in the acute phase (see Case 65). In some patients, however, the early lesion goes unnoticed, particularly in the elderly. This collection becomes walled off by a capsule over a period of a few weeks. The lesion develops an osmotic effect and fluid is drawn in, causing it to swell, thereby producing pressure and distortion of the brain. This may present several weeks after the injury with headache, weakness, dementia, etc., and is an important and potentially curable cause of these symptoms. In common with other fresh bleeds the haematoma is of high density in the acute stage (see Case 16). This density gradually diminishes as the fluid is drawn in, until the collection becomes of lower density than brain. This situation has been reached in the haematoma on the right. The lesion on the left is isodense, however, suggesting that it has developed at a different rate to that on the right. An isodense subdural haematoma may be very difficult to see on plain scans, but there will be effacement of the cortical sulci and evidence of a mass effect. Where such a lesion is suggested by these signs, contrast enhancement may outline the margin of the collection and its interface with brain. Arteriography can also show this lesion by demonstrating displacement of the brain surface away from the vault (see Case 32). Isotope scanning will usually demonstrate vague uptake over the affected hemisphere (see Case 92). In some patients the collection may form layers of different densities (see Case 32). Chronic subdural haematomas can go undiagnosed for years and in such cases the capsule may become calcified. Such a case (again bilateral) is shown below in image C.

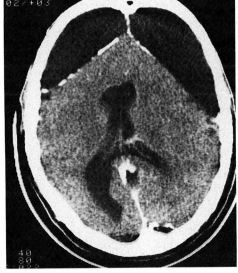

C

Case 8

Male aged 53 years.
Recurrent headache of 4 years' duration.
Mild left-sided weakness.

Q: What abnormalities are present on plain film A?
    What would you do next?

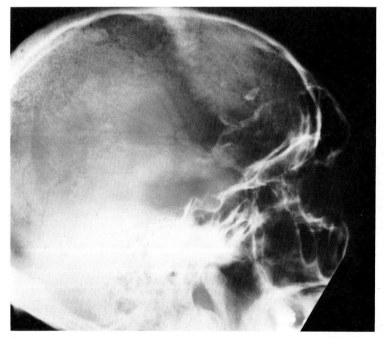

A

Case 8   Oligodendroglioma

This lateral skull film shows two important abnormalities. The dorsum sella and posterior floor of the pituitary fossa are poorly defined suggesting raised intracranial pressure. Irregular calcification is present overlying the frontal lobes. These findings suggest a calcified intracranial mass and further techniques are indicated. MRI does not show calcification well and this sign cannot be properly assessed by this technique, therefore CT is the next most appropriate step. Angiography may be helpful as many vascular lesions show calcification.

The CT scan on this patient is shown below in images B and C. Scan B is unenhanced and shows curved calcification in the right frontal lobe. Scan C following enhancement shows some increased density, most of which is lateral to the calcified area. There is also some low density within the lesion and shift of midline structures to the left.

There are several diagnostic possibilities for a calcified lesion such as this. Low-grade glial tumours such as astrocytoma or oligodendroglioma may calcify and enhancement in these is often unobtrusive. AVMs commonly calcify, but usually show prominent enhancement without mass effect (see Case 9). Furthermore, raised intracranial pressure is not a feature of AVMs. Longstanding granulomas or old abscesses could look like this but there was nothing in the patient's history to suggest these possibilities. Giant aneurysms commonly have calcified walls but usually show intense enhancement within the lumen (see Case 57).

The most likely diagnosis therefore is an astrocytoma or oligodendroglioma. The lesion could be either of these but the heavy calcification and frontal lobe position favours oligodendroglioma. This tumour is one of the least aggressive brain tumours and many patients survive for years with a minimum of surgical intervention. Isotope studies and angiography may show evidence of a tumour of low vascularity, but will not usually provide much help in defining its nature.

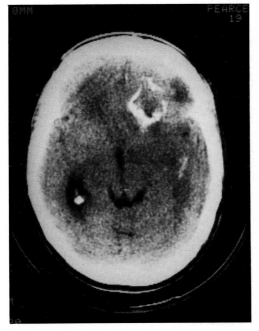

B

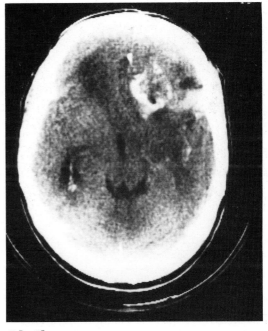

C [+C]

Case 9

Female, aged 59 years.
Recent history of headaches. Mild weakness of left arm
and leg.

Q: These CT images were obtained. What firm
   diagnosis can you make?

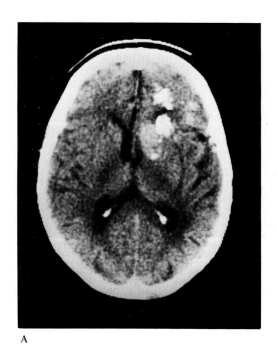

A

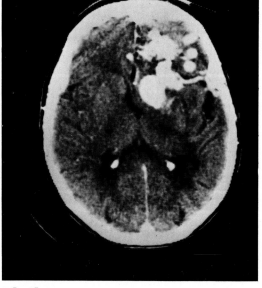

B [+C]

Case 9   Arteriovenous malformation (AVM)

Image A is from an unenhanced CT scan on this
patient and shows areas of mixed raised density in the
right frontal area. The areas of very high density are
into the range of calcification and the less dense areas
are well-defined. There is some widening of the right
Sylvian fissure suggesting local atrophy. Scan B was
taken after contrast enhancement and shows that
those areas, previously of mildly raised density, have
enhanced markedly and show a serpiginous outline.
This latter feature suggests blood vessels and these are
indeed large dilated veins. These appearances are
entirely characteristic of an AVM.

Arteriovenous malformations constitute a spectrum
of abnormal arterial to venous shunts or fistulae. The
shunt may occur at arterial, capillary or venous levels;
of these only direct arterial to venous shunts are
common. These lesions are usually congenital in
origin but can be the result of local trauma. Patients
with such a lesion may present with headaches, fits or a
progressive deficit such as weakness. Around 10 per
cent of all subarachnoid haemorrhages are due to
AVMs and these present in a similar fashion to a
ruptured   aneurysm   (*see*   Case   13).   Wholly
intracerebral haemorrhage from an AVM is also a
common presentation. The possibility of such an
underlying lesion should be kept in mind in any
apparently spontaneous intracerebral haemorrhage
(*see* Case 16).

AVMs can be suspected on plain films of the skull
where the lesion may show calcification or pressure
erosion of adjacent bones. Isotope scans can show
serpiginous   areas   of   high   uptake.   CT   scan
appearances are very characteristic with areas of
calcification, focal atrophy, varying density and
prominent enhancement. Mass effect is rare except in
the   presence   of   recent   haemorrhage.   Such
haemorrhage may obscure the AVM and its presence
may only become evident on follow-up scans or on
angiography. Arteriography is frequently required to
confirm the diagnosis and delineate the associated
vessels so that decisions about possible surgical or
embolic management can be made. Rapid passage of
contrast medium into the venous circulation is
evident; the feeding arteries and draining veins are
enlarged and tortuous. Multiple vessels may have to
be studied to show the entire blood supply to the
lesion. Image C is from this patient's arteriogram and
demonstrates the grossly enlarged and tortuous
draining veins. MRI can provide valuable information
in these cases since blood flow shows characteristic
signal deficits. This technique also appears to be the
best way to demonstrate small slow-flowing fistulae
('cryptic' AVMs).

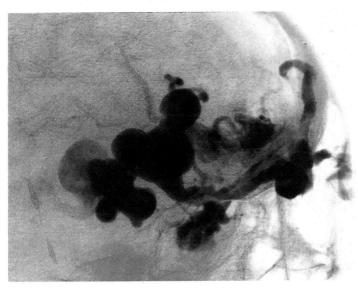

C

Case 10

Male, aged 29 years. Long history of headaches.
Left proptosis and double vision.

Q: Images A and B are plain skull films on this
patient. What do they show?

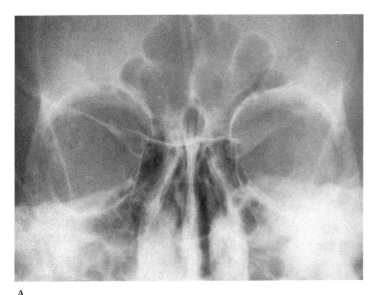

A

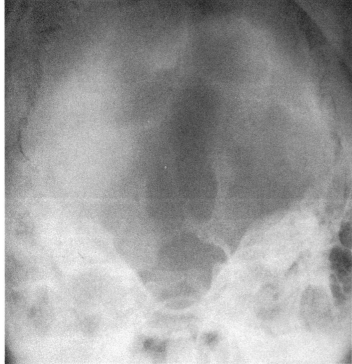

B

Case 10   Neurofibromatosis

The combination of headaches and visual problems constitute a clear indication for further investigation on this patient. Image A is a PA 20° plain film of the skull. This projection is particularly good for demonstration of the bony features of the orbits. The superior orbital fissure is normal on the right side. The fissure on the left is markedly widened and distorted with slight thickening of its well-defined margins. Image B is a Towne's projection on the same patient. This view demonstrates the occipital bone well and this is seen to contain a fairly well-defined, but somewhat irregular area of diminished bone density. These lesions could be caused by several processes including fibrous dysplasia, neurofibromatosis, histiocytosis or metastases. Fibrous dysplasia usually shows bone thickening with areas of increased density and some degree of 'ground-glass' texture (*see Figure 25*). Histiocytosis is encountered in younger patients than this and the bone lesions lack a cortical margin. Metastatic lesions have ill-defined margins in bone.

The appearance in the orbit is very suggestive of neurofibromatosis. This neuroectodermal disorder is characterized by skin changes and an increased incidence of tumours, especially optic glioma, meningioma and neuromas on the acoustic or other cranial nerves. Neuromas on peripheral nerves are also common. The changes seen in the orbit are typical of this condition and are the result of aplasia of the greater wing of sphenoid rather than a neuroma. Exophthalmos is often associated with this bony change. The vault may be asymmetrical and other bony defects may be present as in this case. It was subsequently established that this patient's headaches were due to another unrelated cause and these bony changes were an incidental finding.

An example of a neuromatous mass in the middle cranial fossa producing a lobulated enhancing area extending into the posterior part of the right orbit is shown on CT scanning in image C.

See also optic chiasm glioma (Case 59).

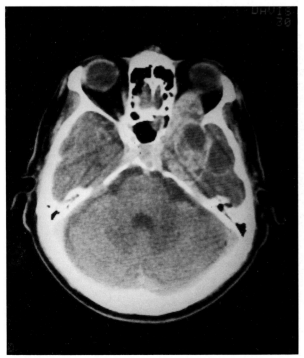

C [+C]

Case 11

Male, aged 42 years.
Intermittent headache. Moderate papilloedema.

Q: The lateral skull film shows a suspicious sign.
    What is it, and what does it suggest?

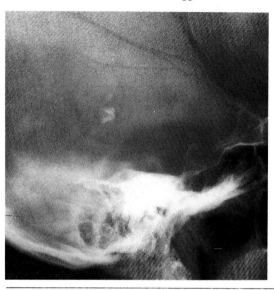

Case 12

Female, aged 50 years.
Vague headaches, often severe, for 2 months.
Varying neurological signs.

Q: What differential diagnosis would you consider
    on the evidence revealed by this enhanced scan?

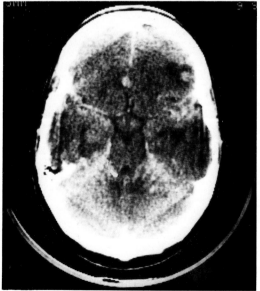

[+C]

Case 11   Pinealoma

This film shows an unusually large calcified pineal gland. When this is more than 1 cm in diameter this finding suggests a tumour of the pineal. Tumours of the pineal gland may be of several histological types, germinoma being the most common. CT shows a mass in the pineal region with a variable amount of calcification and enhancement. Hydrocephalus is invariably present and may be intermittent in character due to obstruction of the posterior third ventricle. In this patient the history of headache was due to the presence of hydrocephalus.

Gliomas, lipomas and true pineal cell tumours also occur in this location.

Case 12   Tuberculous meningitis/granulomas

This CT scan image shows vague increased enhancement along the margins of the tentorium and in the right Sylvian fissure. Small discrete areas of enhancement are also present in the anterior interhemispheral fissure, and inferior lateral aspect of the right frontal lobe. Such changes suggest a pathological process primarily based on the meninges. The possible causes for this appearance include metastatic disease (*see* Case 43), or meningitis due to tuberculosis or other infective organisms including fungi and protozoa. These conditions may also produce focal masses called granulomas and the discrete lesions in this case probably represent small early examples of this. Sarcoidosis can produce a similar appearance. Tuberculous granulomas can be present for many months before the diagnosis is made. Occasionally calcification in the basal cisterns may be seen. In countries where tuberculosis is endemic, some granulomas may show a low-density area with irregular enhancement suggestive of glioma.

Acute headache

General considerations

This section should be read in conjunction with the previous chapter on subacute or recurrent headache. The mechanisms for production of headache have already been described.

Acute headache is a very common complaint and the majority of cases are due to simple and relatively harmless conditions. A first attack of migraine can be a source of considerable concern. The general features of migraine are described in the previous chapter, as is temporal arteritis which usually has a less than acute presentation. Toxic headaches are associated with a variety of conditions such as over-indulgence in alcohol and the fever of viral infections including the childhood exanthemata. Acute sinusitis is suggested by constant unilateral boring pain at the appropriate site; fever is also present. Acute hypertension can present with acute headache; an underlying cause should be sought. None of the foregoing usually require imaging investigations except where atypical features are present.

Acute intracranial infections such as meningitis are characterized by increasing headache, fever and neck stiffness. An abscess will tend to produce localizing neurological signs. Intracranial haemorrhage produces headache by direct irritation of the meninges if the blood is subarachnoid in location, or by distortion of the brain arteries and raised intracranial pressure if the bleed is intracerebral. The headache of subarachnoid haemorrhage is characteristically dramatic in onset and is associated with neck stiffness. Intracerebral bleeds are also of sudden onset and may show neurological deficit appropriate to their location. Acute hydrocephalus, particularly of the type associated with ball-valve obstruction of the CSF pathways by tumour, may be suspected if the acute headache is encountered in particular positions of the head (hydrocephalic 'attacks').

Any acute headache associated with neck stiffness, neurological signs or altered consciousness, or that is posturally provoked merits further investigation by imaging techniques. The plain skull film has little value in management of these cases, except where sinus disease needs to be excluded. CT scanning is the mainstay of diagnosis in acute headache; haemorrhage, encephalitis, abscess, hydrocephalus etc., are usually readily demonstrated and appropriate management can be instituted. Angiography is usually required to further evaluate cases of haemorrhage. MRI can show most of these lesions but has no obvious advantage over CT in the management of these cases.

The following list includes the commoner causes of acute headache with imaging manifestations. The first eight causes are described in the ensuing cases. The other cases are covered elsewhere as they are more usually associated with other presenting symptoms and signs.

Subarachnoid haemorrhage
Intracerebral haemorrhage
Encephalitis
Cerebral abscess
Venous occlusion
Subdural abscess
Meningitis
Acute hydrocephalus
Septic infarction (Case 47)
Cerebral oedema (Case 62)
Arteritis (Case 27)
Cerebral infarction (Case 22)
Acute subdural haematoma (Case 65)
Haemorrhage into tumour (Case 69)
Haemorrhagic infarction (Case 25)

Case 13

Female, aged 34 years.
Sudden onset of severe headache with neck stiffness.
No previous history of headache.

Q: Images A and B were obtained. What is this
   diagnostic technique, and what does it show?
Q: Image C is from the same patient. Why was this
   procedure performed?

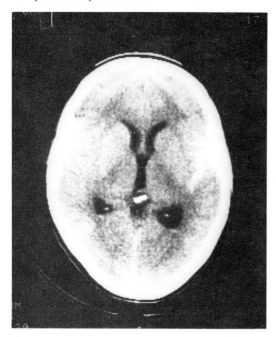

A

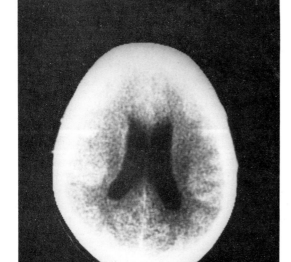

B

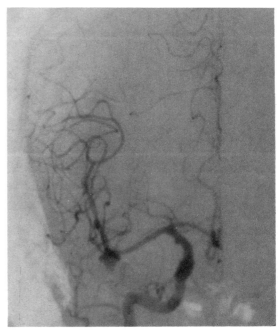

C

Case 13   Subarachnoid haemorrhage (SAH)

Images A and B are from an unenhanced CT scan and show an irregular area of raised density in the right Sylvian fissure. The ventricles are mildly dilated for a patient of this age. This is the typical appearance of fresh blood mixed with CSF in the basal cisterns— subarachnoid haemorrhage.

SAH is a common cause of acute headache. The onset is usually precipitous and may be associated with physical stress. Neck stiffness or photophobia are commonly associated and the CSF is usually blood-stained or xanthochromic on lumbar puncture. Most cases are the result of rupture of a berry aneurysm on the circle of Willis, but other causes such as AVM or tumour may be responsible. The common sites of aneurysms are shown in Diagram D, together with the incidence of aneurysms at each site.

Although the aneurysm can rupture into the cerebral substance, in most instances the blood passes directly into the subarachnoid space where it is diluted by CSF. Because of this dilution the density of the blood on CT is usually significantly less than in intracerebral bleeds (*see* Case 16) and careful scrutiny of the scans may be necessary to confirm this important diagnosis. Furthermore, the dilution causes the blood to clear rapidly (3–6 days) and a scan should be obtained as early as possible to detect it. As a result of its subarachnoid location, the high density tends to follow the position and configuration of the major cisterns. Although often diffuse, it may be localized to the immediate vicinity of the aneurysm. Many cases develop hydrocephalus, mostly as a result of obstruction to CSF pathways by blood which may also be seen within the ventricles. Most aneurysms are too small to be visualized directly on CT and angiography will be required for their demonstration. Image C is an AP film from a right carotid arteriogram on this patient and shows a rounded bulge at the point of division of the right middle cerebral artery. This is the offending aneurysm and many of the vessels are narrowed and irregular due to spasm (*see* Case 26). Surgical clipping of aneurysms produces good results in preventing further bleeds and detailed angiography is required for a full preoperative assessment. About 25 per cent of patients have several aneurysms and the whole intracranial circulation may have to be visualized. In such cases the location of the blood on CT will help to decide which aneurysm has bled.

Other imaging modalities have little to offer in the management of SAH. Larger aneurysms may also bleed but often present as space-occupying lesions (*see* Cases 57 and 83).

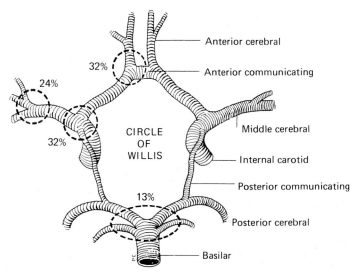

Anterior cerebral

Anterior communicating

32%

24%

Middle cerebral

CIRCLE OF WILLIS

32%

Internal carotid

Posterior communicating

13%

Posterior cerebral

Basilar

D

Case 14

Male aged 27 years.
Sudden onset of severe headache.

Q: This CT scan and arteriogram were obtained.
    How can the low-density area be accounted for?

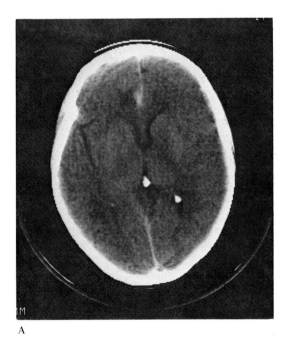

A

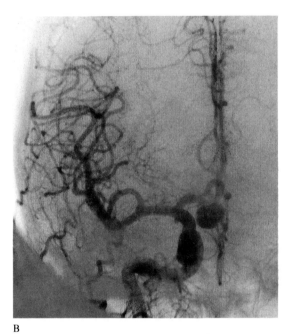

B

Case 14 Subarachnoid haemorrhage

The CT scan shows haemorrhage in the anterior interhemispheral fissure. This subarachnoid blood has come from the anterior communicating artery aneurysm demonstrated on the arteriogram (B). This is another common location for aneurysms. Adjacent to the haemorrhage is an area of low density in the medial aspect of the left frontal lobe. This is probably due to ischaemia as many cases of SAH are associated with arterial spasm (*see* Case 26). This may produce areas of ischaemia or even infarction. By the time this arteriogram was obtained the spasm had passed.

Aneurysms may rupture wholly or partly into the cerebral substance. Image C shows another case with a bleed from an anterior cerebral artery territory aneurysm. In this instance, most of the blood has ruptured into the cerebral substance (in the anterior corpus callosum), and on into the ventricles where it has collected with a horizontal upper surface in the occipital horns. Image D shows generalized SAH in the suprasellar and adjacent cisterns. In this case both temporal horns of the lateral ventricles are also dilated on either side of the haemorrhage-filled cisterns. The source of the haemorrhage is not obvious. SAH may also be seen in the posterior fossa from aneurysms or AVMs on the vertebrobasilar circulation.

When multiple aneurysms are present on angiography and the CT location of SAH is unhelpful, then the largest aneurysm with an irregular outline and associated spasm is usually the source of the bleed.

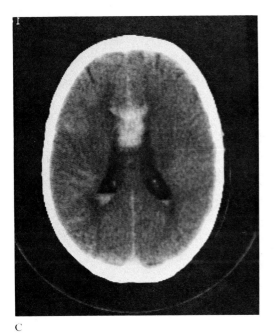

C

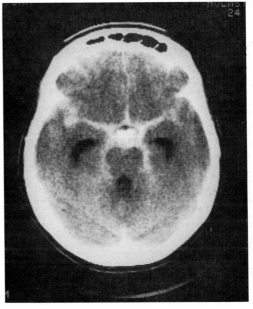

D

Case 15

Female, aged 21 years.
Severe headache for 2 days, mild confusion, moderate fever.
Clinical diagnosis: possible encephalitis.

Q: An immediate CT scan was obtained (A). What does this image show?
Q: What would you do now?

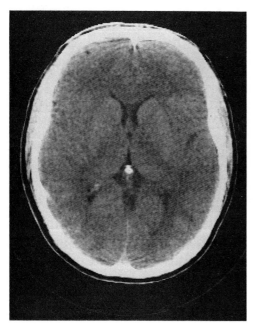

A

Case 15   Acute encephalitis

The scan is quite normal. However, this is not unusual in the early stages of brain infection, particularly in the case of encephalitis, and an early follow-up scan is indicated. When the clinical suspicion is strong and a CT scan is negative, one can proceed to use one of the antiviral agents until the diagnostic appearance is demonstrated on CT, or viral antibody titres confirm the diagnosis.

Encephalitis in Western Europe is usually due to the herpes simplex virus. The presentation is one of headache and fever. Neurological signs such as hemiparesis, cranial nerve palsies, seizures or dysphasia are common. The CT scan is often negative initially but a repeat study 5 or 6 days after the onset will usually show an area of focal oedema in the insula. This is an area of cortex buried by the Sylvian fissure and sharply demarcated medially by the lentiform nucleus. A low-density area here, showing the sharp medial margin with the basal nuclei is very suggestive of encephalitis. This patient showed these changes 10 days later. The unenhanced CT scan then obtained (image B) demonstrated such a lesion in the right insula.

This oedema may spread through the temporal and frontal lobes or show variable enhancement. Follow-up scans may be expected to show focal atrophy. Even the most severely ill patients, however, may continue to have normal scans throughout their illness. (In small children the disease is more severe and there is widespread oedema and, subsequently, necrosis.) Clinically the picture may be very similar to meningitis but the CT changes are very limited in that condition (*see* Case 20). Cerebral abscess shows characteristic enhancement (*see* Case 17), although this feature may not be prominent in the early stages. Venous infarction could show CT changes similar to this but the location and medial margin would be unusual (*see* Case 21). Arterial infarction would be unusual confined to this location (*see* Case 22). Confusion of these appearances with early tumour is possible but careful clinical assessment and sequential scanning should allow differentiation.

It has been claimed that isotope scans will show non-specific uptake in many cases where the CT is still normal. Early experience with MRI suggests that it may also be able to detect the changes sooner than with CT.

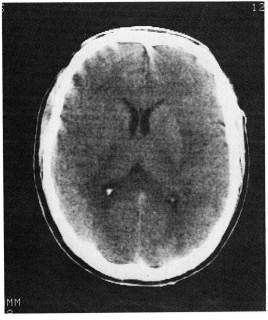

B

Case 16

Female, aged 52 years.
Sudden onset of severe headache, mild right-sided weakness.

Q: What important sign is present on film A?
Q: A CT scan was obtained and is shown in B. What does it show, and how does this relate to the plain-film changes? What other investigation may be required to complete the diagnosis?

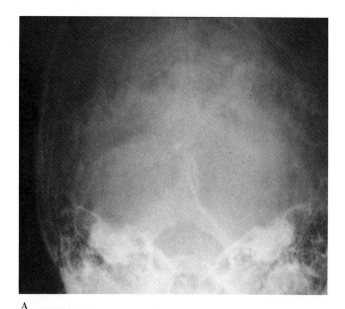

A

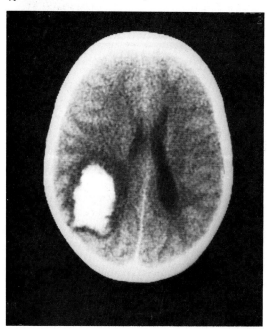

B

Case 16   Intracerebral haemorrhage (AVM)

The AP skull film shows a calcified pineal gland which is displaced to the right side. This finding, together with the right-sided weakness, is consistent with a space-occupying process in the left hemisphere. The CT scan confirms this and shows an irregular high-density lesion in the upper left parietal lobe. The lesion is surrounded by a rim of low-density oedema and there is compression of the left lateral ventricle, with both ventricles displaced to the right. This latter feature confirms the midline shift shown on the plain film.

The appearances are those of an intracerebral haemorrhage. Patients may present with headache, sudden coma or a variety of neurological deficits, such as hemiplegia, depending on the location of the bleed. Neck stiffness may occur if a subarachnoid component is present. The causes of bleeding into the cerebral substance are legion but the more important include hypertension, aneurysm, arteriovenous malformation, trauma, tumours, bleeding disorders and ischaemia. These conditions are discussed in various cases throughout the book under other clinical presentations and the reader is referred to the pathology index at the end of the book.

The CT appearance of a high-density lesion surrounded by a low-density zone (due to oedema or clot retraction) is fairly typical of intracerebral haemorrhage. Calcification can have this appearance but the acute story is against this. In cases of difficulty an assessment of numerical values of density will usually resolve the problem, as calcification shows values of 100 Hounsfield units or more, while haemorrhage has a density of 50–70 units. Fresh haemorrhage has a high protein content and is of higher density than brain tissue, producing these changes on CT. Over a few days or weeks the haemorrhage is resorbed and the density fades. Enhancement may show an underlying lesion such as a tumour or AVM, but the density of the blood often obscures this pattern in the early days. A follow-up CT scan when the density has cleared, or an arteriogram, will help to exclude such underlying lesions. Hypertensive haemorrhage usually occurs in the basal nuclei and does not normally require further evaluation. Haemorrhage elsewhere, unless the result of trauma, may need additional assessment. An arteriogram was obtained on this patient and showed a small AVM in the left parietal area which was successfully excised (image C). A spontaneous cerebellar haemorrhage is shown in D.

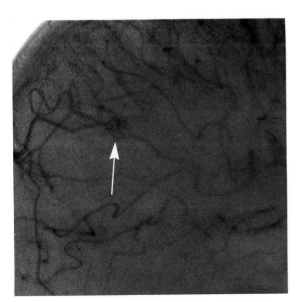

C

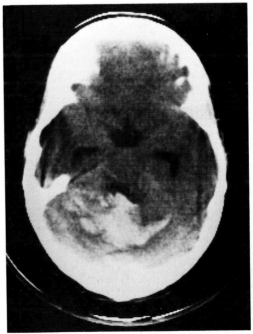

D

Case 17

Female, aged 50 years.
Severe headache of several days' duration, increasing confusion and fever.
Because of the increasing confusion a CT scan was obtained to exclude encephalitis. The unenhanced CT scan (A) shows a low-density area in the right temporal lobe. The enhanced scan (B) shows a ring of enhancement in this area.

Q: What lesion might this be, and what is the relevance of the plain film (C)?

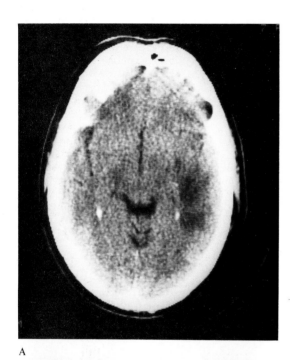

A

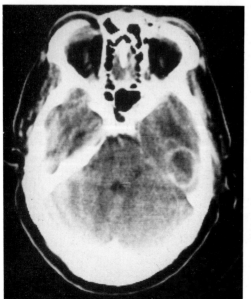

B [+C]

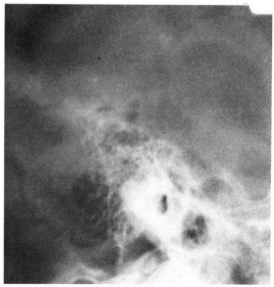

C

Case 17   Cerebral abscess

The CT appearances are consistent with a cerebral abscess. This condition is a serious neurological emergency and early diagnosis is essential if there is to be an opportunity for a satisfactory outcome.

Clinical diagnosis is often difficult as fever may be absent. The CT scan can be the first occasion at which the possibility is raised. During the first few days an abscess may simply show an area of non-specific focal cerebral oedema such as is seen on scan A. The enhancing ring may not be evident at this stage until a capsule starts to form. A definitive diagnosis cannot be made on CT until this ring is demonstrated. The ring is usually circular, or nearly so, and has a thin regular margin. Similar appearances may be seen in metastases, gliomas, resolving haematoma or granulomas, but rarely do these show such a thin regular ring, and the acute onset with fever is also against these diagnoses.

Most cerebral abscesses are associated with infection in the middle ear, sinusitis or septicaemia, and such a source must be sought with diligence. Plain film C is a view of the right mastoid bone in this patient. Compare this image with that in *Figure 8* of a normal mastoid appearance. In this present patient, the mastoid air cells are opaque due to acute mastoiditis—the source of infection for this patient's cerebral abscess. Such ear or sinus infections may lead to other intracranial problems such as venous thrombosis (*see* Case 21) or subdural abscesses (*see* Case 19).

Abscesses are not uncommonly multiple (*see* image D). These are usually embolic in origin, perhaps due to cardiac disease. Isotope scanning will show an abscess as an area of increased uptake but the appearances are non-specific. Angiography may show abnormal vessels and a general pattern very difficult to differentiate from malignant tumour circulation. The role of MRI in the management of cerebral abscess is as yet undetermined, but early studies suggest it may facilitate earlier diagnosis of the abscess structure.

A cerebral abscess may rupture into the subdural space and produce a subdural abscess (*see* Case 19), or into the ventricular system to produce ventriculitis. In this situation the CSF may be denser than usual due to the presence of pus, and the ependyma may show enhancement due to hyperaemia. Image E shows these changes in the left lateral ventricle of a patient where an abscess just above the left trigone has ruptured into the ventricle to produce unilateral ventriculitis.

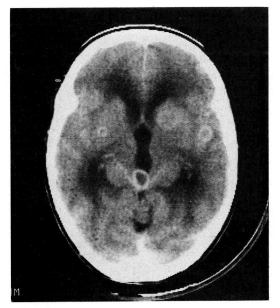

D [+C]

E [+C]

Case 18

Female, aged 37 years.
Sudden onset of severe headache while bending forward.
Previous episode 8 months before.

Q: This CT scan was obtained without enhancement. The appearances are highly suggestive of what specific diagnosis?

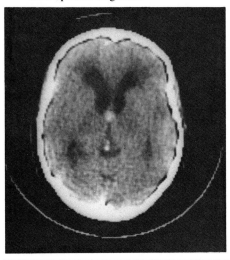

Case 19

Male, aged 16 years.
Increasing headache for 5 days, now semi-comatose and feverish.

Q: Images A and B are from a CT scan on this patient. What do they show, and can you identify the lesions on the plain scan?

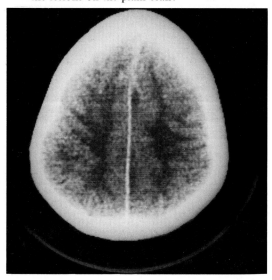

A

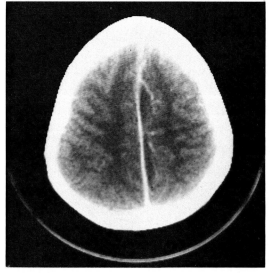

B [+C]

Case 18   Colloid cyst

A history of sudden severe headache can indicate the presence of a lesion within the ventricular system causing acute obstruction by a ball-valve type of action. These bouts of obstruction can be brief and they may be precipitated by placing the head in certain positions. A possible cause is an intraventricular tumour.

The CT scan shows a high-density lesion in the anterior part of the third ventricle with some dilatation of the lateral ventricles. These appearances are almost diagnostic of a colloid cyst of the third ventricle. This tumour is a benign cyst filled with a colloidal material. It invariably arises in this site where it produces obstruction to the foramina of Munro with resultant dilatation of the lateral ventricles, while the third ventricle is of normal size or small. The colloidal contents are usually of higher density than surrounding brain but occasionally the lesion is isodense, in which case it's presence can only be inferred from obliteration of the anterior third ventricle.

Other lesions which may be found within the ventricular system leading to obstruction include, pinealoma (*see* Case 11), ependymoma (*see* Case 80), choroid plexus papilloma (*see* Case 42), glioma and meningioma (*see* Case 28).

Case 19   Subdural abscess

Plain scan A shows vague swelling or oedema in both upper hemispheres. This appearance is non-specific and should arouse considerable suspicion as this plain-scan finding may reflect a wide variety of intracranial pathology. This includes subdural haematoma or abscess, venous occlusion, etc. Where such a vague change is seen on a plain scan it is best to pursue further information with contrast enhancement. Scan B shows curvilinear enhancement along the right side of the falx. These lines delineate shallow low-density areas, which in retrospect are just visible on the plain scan. These areas are very suggestive of subdural abscesses. This is an unusual intracranial infection where the pus collects in pockets along the subdural space. These collections may be found anywhere over the surface of the brain and may be very difficult to see when situated along the base, or the tentorium. Most cases are due to spread from sources similar to those of abscesses within the brain substance (*see* Case 17), others result from an infected subdural haematoma. Subdural abscesses are commonly multiple and carry a poor prognosis. They can be very difficult to diagnose clinically and may also be missed on CT if contrast enhancement is not given. The principal differential diagnosis on CT is chronic subdural haematoma, but this lesion is not associated with fever and is less localized.

Case 20

Female, aged 23 years.
Marked headache for 3 days. Some photophobia.
Marked neck stiffness and fever.

Q: It was felt important to exclude encephalitis although there was no evidence of impaired consciousness. CT scanning was not available and an isotope study was normal. Images A and B are from the arteriogram. What do they show?

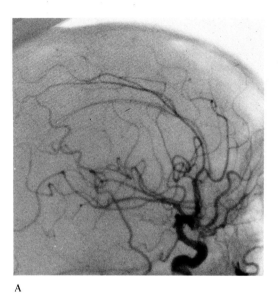

A

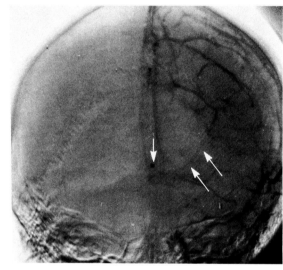

B

Case 21

Female aged 22 years.
Severe headache and mild confusion for 4 days.
On oral contraceptives.

Q: A CT scan showed only vague cerebral oedema and an angiogram was obtained. Image A is an oblique film in the venous phase. Image B is a normal study for comparison. What abnormality is shown?

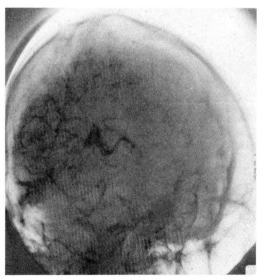

A

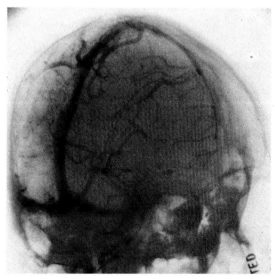

B

Case 20   Hydrocephalus due to meningitis

Image A is a lateral film from the arteriogram during the arterial phase. The curve of the pericallosal artery is considerably widened (*compare with Figure 54*). This may be due to its being displaced by midline shift, or by hydrocephalus. Image B shows an AP view of the venous phase, the internal cerebral vein is not displaced to either side so there is no midline shift (short arrow). The thalamostriate vein (long arrows) outlines the lateral margin of the ventricle which is obviously enlarged (*compare with Figure 57*). The arteriographic findings are consistent with hydrocephalus. This is an important but non-specific finding with a wide variety of causes. In this case the patient had meningitis, previously confirmed by analysis of CSF after lumbar puncture. Inflammation of the meninges often has no radiological manifestations but may cause obstruction to CSF pathways. In patients with signs of raised intracranial pressure hydrocephalus may have to be excluded by CT or other studies before a confirmatory lumbar puncture is performed. MRI may show areas of 'infarction' in the peripheral cortex in some cases of meningitis. These may be the result of local microvascular damage related to the thickened meninges.

Case 21   Venous occlusion

In the normal study (B), the large curved structure superiorly is the superior sagittal sinus. Within this curve, at its centre, is a much smaller but similarly curved structure—the internal cerebral vein (*see Angiographic anatomy in Part I*). This patient's venous phase film shows only the internal cerebral vein and the small cortical veins (A). The superior sagittal sinus is not filling because it is thrombosed.

Intracranial venous thrombosis is common and may be associated with generalized systemic infections, oral contraception, dehydration or direct involvement of venous sinuses by fractures, tumours, etc. Clinical presentation is variable but haemorrhagic infarction is common (*see Case 25*). Vague areas of low-density or generalized oedema may also be seen on CT. Dynamic isotope studies may be helpful to demonstrate occluded sinuses. MRI can also show changes in the flow voids normally seen in the venous sinuses but artefacts can make assessment difficult. Angiography is required in many cases for a definitive diagnosis, especially where only a few cortical veins are involved.

Sudden unilateral weakness

General considerations

The sudden onset of weakness of one or both limbs on one side of the body is a common clinical presentation, and will invariably lead to further investigation. Weakness principally affecting cranial nerve muscles is covered in the chapter dealing with disorders of those structures. Limb weakness of long duration or of gradual onset is dealt with in the next section, p. 117.

Sudden unilateral weakness implies an acute lesion of the motor fibres between the cerebral cortex and the muscles controlling the affected limb. Lesions in peripheral nerves are characterized by lower motor neurone signs and are not covered here. Limb weakness arising from spinal cord lesions is rarely unilateral and is usually accompanied by characteristic sensory signs. Any acute lesion affecting the motor cortex in the precentral area is likely to produce a corresponding weakness on the opposite side of the body. The lesion may be quite small and only one limb, or a part of it, is then affected. The motor fibres descend through the internal capsule where, because the fibres are closely grouped, a small lesion produces a very extensive neurological deficit. The fibres pass on through the midbrain into the brainstem, and then to the cervical cord. Lesions within the motor tract, or causing the relevant structures to be distorted or compressed, can produce unilateral weakness. At these levels other structures are also usually involved, and hydrocephalus, cranial nerve deficits or other posterior fossa symptoms or signs may provide important clinical evidence about the level in the brain at which the lesion has occurred.

A wide variety of pathology can affect the motor tracts. However, the possibilities are somewhat more limited when the onset is sudden; migraine, temporal arteritis or multiple sclerosis may all produce hemiparesis of sudden onset, and usually there is little to be seen on imaging techniques, although there is a need for thorough investigation to exclude some other cause. In the first two conditions, intracranial vessels are occluded by spasm or inflammation to produce the deficit; vague areas of ischaemia may be seen on CT. In multiple sclerosis the lesion is an acute demyelinating plaque and this may be visualized on MRI using T2-weighted sequences. MRI is abnormal in nearly all cases subsequently shown to have MS. Transient ischaemic attacks produce neurological deficits of 24 hours' duration or less and are followed by complete resolution; hemiparesis is one of the common presentations and the cause is usually embolic; CT is invariably normal but serves to exclude other pathology. In selected cases angiography may be required (*see* Case 48).

The major causes of acute hemiparesis include infarction and intracerebral haemorrhage. Characteristically of sudden onset, the deficit is sustained for several days or weeks and may be permanent. Some patients are hypertensive or give a history of previous attacks. Headache may be a prominent feature and consciousness or other modalities may be impaired depending on the site and extent of the lesion. For most patients diagnostic imaging is indicated. Plain skull films are usually unhelpful and CT is the most productive technique. This usually determines whether or not a haemorrhage is present. Haemorrhage, even in conjunction with infarction, is a contraindication to anticoagulation. The demonstration of infarction is also usually fairly straightforward and appropriate anticoagulation or antiplatelet measures can be instituted. A diagnosis of haemorrhage or infarction may need to be further defined by angiography, particularly if emergency surgery is being considered. The role of MRI in these conditions has not yet been established, but it is likely that CT will remain the investigation of choice, especially in the acute stage.

Infective processes are usually slower in their development but encephalitis can produce weakness of quite rapid onset. CT may be normal in the early stages but delayed studies should help to differentiate this possibility from evolving infarction. Arteritis, venous infarction or septic embolic disease can be very elusive diagnoses; sequential CT and detailed angiography may be needed. Trauma can be an important cause of sudden weakness. The nature of the insult is usually obvious and an intracerebral haematoma, focal oedema or extradural haematoma at an appropriate site (e.g., over the motor cortex) will usually be evident on CT.

The following list includes the most likely causes of acute unilateral weakness that have imaging manifestations. The first six causes are described on the ensuing pages, the other lesions are described elsewhere under different clinical presentations.

Middle cerebral infarction
Anterior cerebral infarction
Spontaneous intracerebral haemorrhage
Arterial spasm
Arteritis
Haemorrhagic infarction
Haemorrhage into tumour/AVM (Case 69)
Venous infarction (Case 21)
Septic infarction (Case 47)
Encephalitis (Case 15)
Brainstem haemorrhage (Case 68)
Brainstem infarction (Case 85)
Multiple sclerosis (Case 70)
Extradural haematoma (Case 66)

Case 22

Male, aged 58 years.
Sudden-onset dense left hemiplegia.

Q: These two studies were obtained. What is the
relationship between the abnormalities shown on
them?

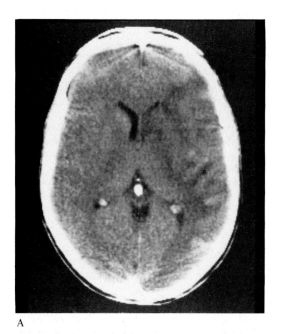

A

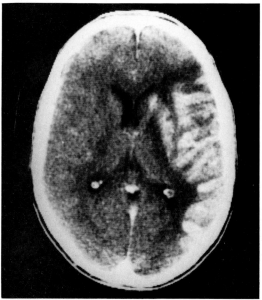

B [+C]

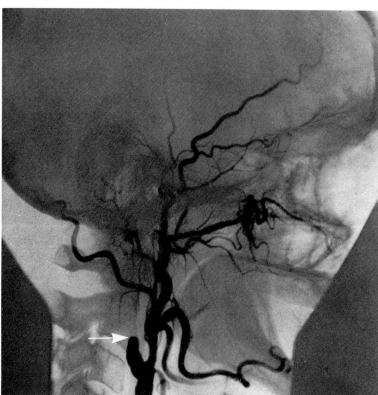

C

Case 22   Infarction: middle cerebral artery territory

Image A is an unenhanced CT scan on this patient. This shows an ill-defined low-density area in the right cerebral hemisphere. This has a wedge-shaped distribution between the frontal horn anteriorly and the ventricular trigone posteriorly. The affected area extends deeply into the basal nuclei and internal capsule, but the thalamus is not involved. There is no mass effect. Image B is an enhanced scan at a slightly higher level and shows prominent enhancement along the lateral margin of the lesion. This has the form of finger-like processes. The appearances are typical of acute infarction in the territory of the middle cerebral artery.

Infarction is a form of tissue necrosis resulting from a major disruption of its blood supply. The shape and size of the tissue involved is dependent on the size and number of vessels involved, and on the extent to which other vessels can sustain blood supply to the whole area. Affected areas are broadly wedge-shaped and these may be quite small and peripherally placed, as in Case 75. Larger lesions follow the configuration of the area of brain supplied by each of the major intracranial vessels. A diagram of these territories is included in the discussion of Case 24. The present case conforms to the pattern of total infarction of the middle cerebral artery territory. An example of incomplete involvement is shown in Case 29. This infarct is usually due to occlusion of the internal carotid artery by atheroma and thrombosis. Although this can lead to complete infarction of the entire hemisphere, the anterior and posterior cerebral territories usually remain perfused via the circle of Willis, but the middle cerebral is insufficiently perfused and infarction results. Depending on the extent to

which circulation is restored either by resolution of the causative block, or collateral supply via other pathways, then the ischaemia may be transient or incomplete. The striking enhancement seen in this case is a common finding in acute infarction and represents increased perfusion along the margins of the ischaemic area, and breakdown of the blood–brain barrier. There is some evidence to suggest that in the first 5–7 days after the onset of infarction this enhancement is harmful and may prejudice long-term recovery. Consequently enhancement is best avoided during this period where infarction is suspected. Further discussion of this important and common condition is given in Cases 24 and 74.

In this case an arteriogram was obtained and is shown in images C and D. Image C is a lateral film in the arterial phase. This shows occlusion of the right internal carotid artery (arrow) shortly after its point of origin from the common carotid artery. At this stage only the branches of the external carotid artery are filled. Image D, taken shortly after C, shows that the external carotid circulation has formed a collateral circulation with the ophthalmic artery and reverse flow in this vessel (short arrow) has filled the carotid siphon enabling faint opacification of the middle cerebral vessels to occur (arrows). Such collateral supplies are common and may occur across the circle of Willis from the other hemisphere or from the posterior fossa. Meningeal branches of the external carotid may also provide collateral supply. Small cortical vessels along the edge of the infarct may also enable collateral flow from adjacent well-perfused tissue to enter the ischaemic area.

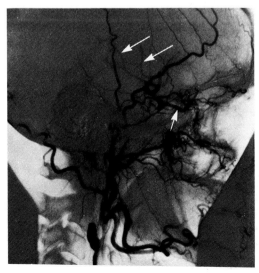

D

Case 23

Female, aged 61 years.
Sudden onset of severe headache and left hemiplegia.
Hypertensive for several years.

Q: What does this CT scan show, and what influence
      does this have on the patient's management?

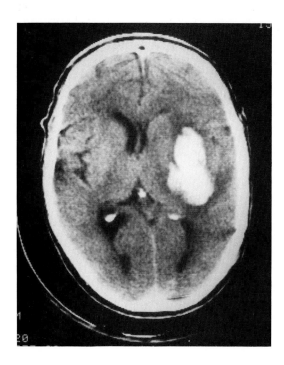

Case 23   Hypertensive haemorrhage

This plain CT scan shows a large haemorrhage involving the right basal nuclei and the internal capsule. There was no change after contrast enhancement. Calcification could look like this but the measured units would be of higher density and the sudden onset also suggests a dramatic vascular lesion. Freshly extravasated blood shows as an area of higher density on CT (*see* Case 16). This finding is very important in this case since the clinical presentation could also be the result of cerebral infarction. Headache, however, is not a prominent feature of infarction. The demonstration of haemorrhage is important since it would be a contraindication to the use of anticoagulants in cases where an infarct was suspected.

Spontaneous intracerebral haemorrhage without an underlying cause such as aneurysm, AVM or trauma is common in hypertensive patients. Most occur in the basal nuclei or brainstem and can produce marked neurological deficits. When spontaneous haemorrhages are encountered in other locations or when the clinical features are suspicious, the possibility of an underlying lesion must be considered. Such a lesion may or may not be evident on the plain scan or after enhancement. Follow-up CT scans when the haemorrhage density has subsided may be more helpful, and angiography may be needed for a full assessment in cases where the underlying lesion might be suitable for treatment. Associated subarachnoid haemorrhage may indicate that the intracerebral haemorrhage is due to aneurysm.

Haemorrhages due to other causes and in other sites are discussed in several other cases, especially 16, 64 and 76.

Case 24

Male, aged 57 years.
Sudden onset of left-sided weakness, most marked in
the leg, 12 days previously.

Q: These CT scans were obtained and considered to
     represent a pattern of recent infarction. Which
     vascular territory do you think is involved?

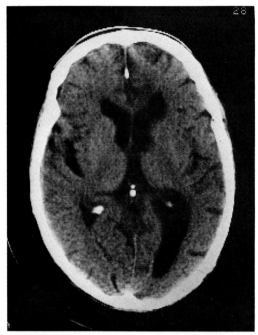

A

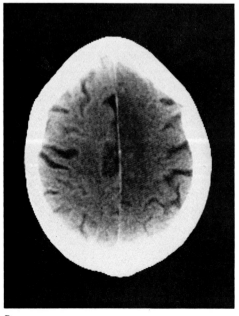

B

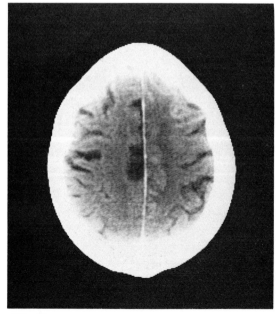

C [+C]

Case 24   Infarction: anterior cerebral artery territory

Scan A is unenhanced and shows a vague low-density area anterior and medial to the frontal horn of the right lateral ventricle. This low density was present on the next superior slice and continuous with a long strip of low density running above the ventricle and adjacent to the falx on scan B. The enhanced scan C shows faint irregular enhancement along the medial aspect of this strip and further enhancement lateral to it anteriorly. This configuration of low density conforms to the distribution of branches of the right anterior cerebral artery. Occlusion of this vessel or its major branches produces an appearance of this kind, and weakness principally affecting the lower limb. Infarction in this territory is less common than in the middle or posterior cerebral arteries. The broad distribution of these three major vascular territories is shown below in D. Partial lesions are commoner than those affecting the full territory. Examples of middle cerebral infarction are shown in Cases 22 and 37. Posterior cerebral artery infarcts are described in Case 74.

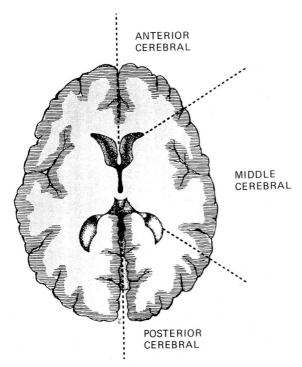

ANTERIOR
CEREBRAL

MIDDLE
CEREBRAL

POSTERIOR
CEREBRAL

D

Case 25

Male, aged 65 years.
Sudden onset of right-sided hemiplegia.

Q: What does this study show?

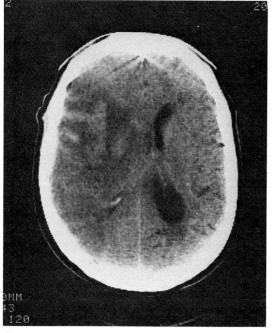

A

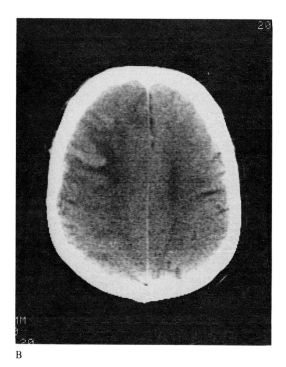

B

Case 25   Haemorrhagic infarction

These unenhanced CT scans show an area of raised density within an area of lower density. The lower density area has a distribution similar to that of infarction in the middle cerebral artery territory. A mass effect is present. This lesion is a combination of haemorrhage and infarction. These haemorrhagic changes may be evident at the onset of the infarct. In some cases, however, they may only be seen several days later within a previously wholly low-density infarct. This process represents a variant of the infarction process described in Case 22. Presumably the occluding embolus moves more distally, allowing blood to enter necrotic vessels within the infarct, which then bleed. In some cases bleeding probably occurs from substitute circulation at the margins of the infarct. Like pure cerebral haemorrhage, the finding of blood within an infarcted area is important as it is a contraindication to the use of anticoagulants in stroke management. About 5–10 per cent of infarcts may show haemorrhagic changes. The combination of haemorrhage and infarction may also be seen as a result of septic emboli (see Case 47), or where infarction is of venous origin (see Case 21).

Infarction of any type may be visible on isotope scanning. The changes are often not marked but conform to vascular territories; they may take a week or more to appear. Serial dynamic studies may confirm major changes to cerebral perfusion. A lateral image from a static isotope series is shown below (image C). A wedge-shaped area of mildly increased uptake in the middle cerebral territory is due to an infarct. This technique is now little used in the assessment of this disease.

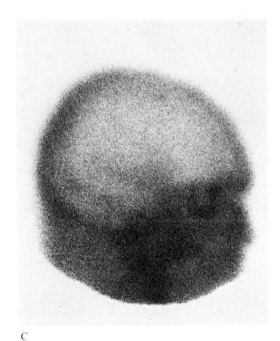

C

Case 26

Male, aged 43 years.
Right-sided weakness.
Severe headache 8 days previously.

Q: What does this arteriogram show, and what is the
relevance of the headache?

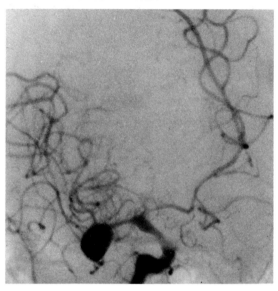

Case 27

Female, aged 19 years.
Right-sided weakness for 3 days.
Mild confusion and dysphasia.

Q: This arteriogram shows an abnormality of the
small arteries (arrows). A CT scan was normal.
What diagnostic possibilities would you
consider?

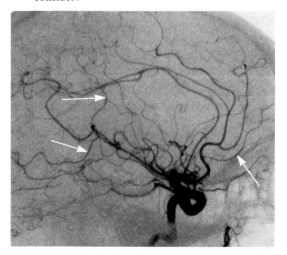

Case 26   Arterial spasm following subarachnoid haemorrhage

This arterial-phase film has been taken in an oblique projection. A CT scan had been normal. The proximal arteries show extensive areas of narrowing. This appearance is typical of arterial spasm. The most likely cause for these changes is SAH (*see* Case 13). Spasm is a common sequel to blood in the CSF and appears 3–10 days after the bleed. The spasm may result in areas of ischaemia or even infarction and there may be changes appropriate to this on the CT scan. Such compromise of the circulation can lead to weakness, dysphasia, confusion, etc. In this case the preceding headache was due to an SAH, but this was not evident on CT since so many days had elapsed since the event (*see* Case 13). A lumbar puncture revealed xanthochromia and angiography was performed. Generalized arterial spasm was present and the aneurysm is shown on the middle cerebral artery.

Case 27   Arteritis

This arteriogram film shows small areas of irregularity in these peripheral arteries. These appearances are unlike spasm which is most evident in the larger arteries at the skull base. Certain tumours cause encasement of small blood vessels but there is no displacement of these vessels or tumour circulation to suggest this diagnosis. In any event one would expect to see evidence of a tumour on the CT scan. Atheroma might cause such irregularities but it would be most unusual to find it so peripherally placed and in such a young patient.

A patient of this age presenting with ischaemia or infarction should be suspected of having a cardiac source of embolism, or arteritis. This latter condition is an inflammatory affection of the cranial arteries. It may accompany a variety of systemic infections and collagen diseases including polyarteritis nodosa and systemic lupus.

Other causes of arteritis which may be encountered include Moya-Moya disease, which produces occlusion of the carotid arteries and extensive collaterals along the base of the brain, and Takayasu's disease affecting the major vessels as they arise from the aortic arch.

Unilateral weakness of gradual onset

General considerations

This section should be read in conjunction with the preceding chapter on hemiparesis of sudden onset. The discussion here deals with weakness of one or both limbs on the same side that has been present for many years or has been developing gradually. Weakness in the distribution of cranial nerves affecting ocular, facial, or tongue movement are dealt with in the section on the posterior fossa and cranial nerves.

The mechanism by which such weakness occurs is very similar to that described in the preceding chapter introduction. The reader is referred to the descriptions given there of the relevant applied anatomy of the motor tracts. As in acute hemiparesis, the lesion is placed on the opposite side of the brain and the power deficit is of the upper motor neurone type, with increased reflexes and no significant muscle wasting. Once again, a careful history and examination will distinguish intracranial causes from those occurring in the spine or peripheral nerves.

Limb weakness of gradual onset or long duration may be produced by many differing pathologies. A variety of vascular, inflammatory, neoplastic, post-traumatic or developmental conditions may be responsible. In many cases there will be other clinical signs resulting from associated raised intracranial pressure: hydrocephalus, seizures, cranial nerve signs or impairment of intellect or consciousness. These features can provide valuable confirmatory evidence that a serious lesion is present, together with indications as to its location and nature. As a group, these lesions have a broad spectrum of appearances on imaging techniques. Plain skull films may be helpful, revealing evidence of raised intracranial pressure, pineal shift, intracranial calcification, vault deformity or relevant bony pathology such as the enostosis of meningioma. A chest radiograph should always be obtained as it may show crucial information regarding primary or secondary neoplasms in the lung, or infective lesions. Such findings may greatly simplify the decision regarding the nature of an unidentified intracranial lesion. CT scanning will reveal most of the underlying causes. Isotope scans may be helpful where CT is not available or for further elucidation of CT appearances. Angiography may be helpful in distinguishing between certain tumours and for further delineation of vascular lesions. MRI scanning may have a valuable contribution in white matter diseases and in lesions below the tentorium.

The causes of longstanding or gradual unilateral weakness are many, and since a significant proportion of them will present in other ways, it has only been possible to cover some of the probable causes in this chapter. The other cases are described elsewhere under other clinical presentations.

Progressive infarction
Established infarction
Malignant astrocytoma
Parasagittal meningioma
Low-grade infection and granuloma e.g. tuberculosis or toxoplasmosis
Leucodystrophy and related disorders
AVM
Chronic subdural haematoma
Intracranial tumours of all types
Hemiatrophy (Case 51)
Previous haemorrhage (Case 76)
Metastases (Case 3)
Intracranial cysts (Case 44)

Case 28

Male, aged 50 years.
Two-year history of weakness of left arm and leg.

Q: What diagnostic technique is this, from what
    aspect of the head was it obtained and what does
    it show?

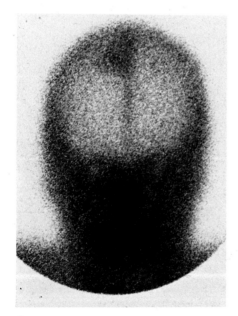

A

Case 28   Parasagittal meningioma

This is an isotope brain scan, and a line of uptake along the falx is clearly visible indicating that the image has been taken either from the anterior or posterior position. The orbits can also be seen signifying that the view must have been taken from the front (anterior). An area of markedly increased uptake is present close to the vertex, just to the right of the falx. The intensity and location of the uptake is highly suggestive of a meningioma in the parasagittal area.

Image B shows the enhanced CT scan in this patient. A well-defined area of enhancement is present adjacent to the falx on the right-hand side. Its appearance is also consistent with a meningioma. This is one of the common locations in which meningiomas occur. They may arise from the falx or from the adjacent convexity. Their presence may go unnoticed for some time unless, as in this case, the lesion presses on a sensitive area of brain such as the motor cortex. Meningiomas in this location may invade and occlude the superior sagittal sinus. This important fact (for the surgeon) can be demonstrated by disruption of flow patterns in the sinus as visualized on MRI. Where MRI is not available, angiography with late films of the venous phase will usually demonstrate this complication. Larger lesions can penetrate the vault and produce extensive bone erosion and sclerosis.

Image C shows a further meningioma lying within the ventricle. This lesion is rare but usually found, as here, at the trigone. It may be very difficult to distinguish it from lymphoma (see Case 93), or choroid plexus papilloma (see Case 42). Other manifestations of meningiomas are discussed in Cases 2 and 72.

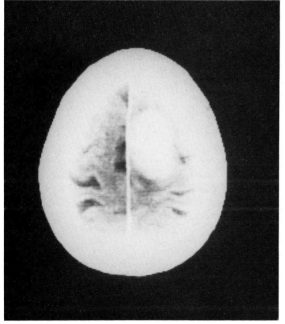

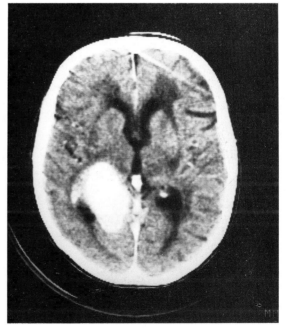

B [+C]   C [+C]

Case 29

Female, aged 49 years.
Slowly progressive right-sided weakness over 1 week.

Q: The CT scan in image A was obtained the day
    after the patient presented. Image B shows the
    appearance 8 days later. What is your diagnosis?
    What other investigations might be required?

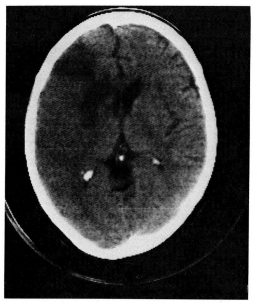

A

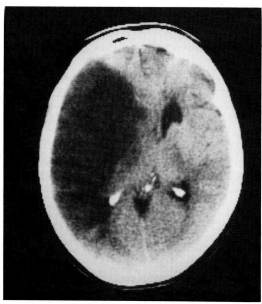

B

Case 29   Progressive infarction

This case provides a graphic demonstration of the value of serial CT scanning in the elucidation of diagnostic problems. The first scan shows low-density areas in the left anterior internal capsule and more peripherally in the cortex where the defect is wedge-shaped. Contrast enhancement was not given as it was felt that the lesions probably represented infarcts and there is evidence to suggest that contrast enhancement in the early phase of infarction may be harmful.

Image B, also without contrast enhancement, shows that the lesions are now part of a large low-density area having the configuration of the territory of the middle cerebral artery. There is also marked midline shift. This latter feature is somewhat unusual in infarction but the configuration of the lesion is typical. This lesion has progressed too rapidly to be a tumour. Encephalitis is also a possibility but the initial site is

against this (*see* Case 15) and there was no history of headache.

Angiography might be helpful to confirm occlusion of the middle cerebral artery or several of its branches. The lenticulostriate branches are probably partly spared in this case as the basal nuclei anteriorly are not completely involved. The source is likely to be atheroma in the internal carotid artery with or without a complete block of that vessel (*see* Case 22).

A further CT scan 3 weeks later is shown in image C. The mass effect has now largely subsided and the configuration of the lesion is typical of middle cerebral infarction. A low-density area is also present in front of the right frontal horn, suggesting a small infarct in the anterior cerebral artery territory on this side.

An infarct of this size is likely to produce long-term hemiparesis. In some cases early scans can be normal.

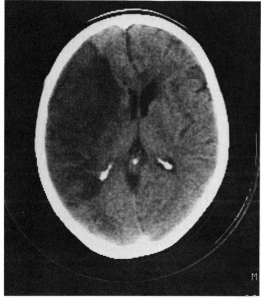

C

Case 30

Female, aged 36.
Nine-month history of slowly progressive left-sided weakness.

Q: The plain film and CT scan below were obtained.
      What do they show?

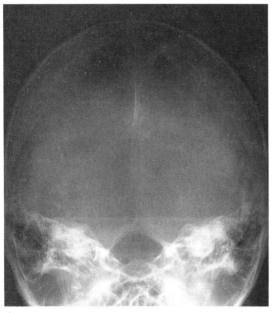

A

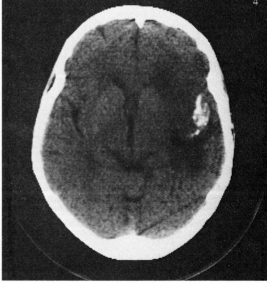

B

Case 30   Malignant astrocytoma

The plain film, which is a Towne's projection, shows calcification projected above the right petrous bone. This could be at several sites in the sagittal plane, including the cerebellum, temporal lobe, etc. A lateral film showed that it lay in the temporal region. The pineal is not calcified so it is not possible to assess shift. The CT scan confirms the presence of calcification in the right temporal area. Behind this, and in front of it, are areas of varying low density. There is very slight distortion of the adjacent ventricle and early shift. There was no change after contrast enhancement.

The differential diagnoses of intracranial calcification are legion. This is not a site for physiological calcification, so some pathological process is present. Aneurysms, old abscesses, etc. may calcify, as can areas of previous tumour, radiotherapy or surgery. There was no history of any such process, however, and the absence of enhancement makes meningioma or aneurysm unlikely. Some benign tumours calcify, notably oligodendroglioma and astrocytoma. The latter was felt to be the most likely and for a variety of reasons nothing further was done at that stage.

Four months later the patient presented again with more rapid deterioration and papilloedema was found to be present. A repeat CT scan was obtained (image C). This has been enhanced and shows a very considerable mass effect on the right, with gross midline shift to the left and compression of the right lateral ventricle. The calcified area is now associated with an area of enhancement.

It seems likely that the original lesion had been present for some time and was originally a low-grade astrocytoma. It has been known for tumours to change their degree of malignancy over a period of time. The long story in this case, with more rapid deterioration, would fit with this, and the change in appearance of the scan is also consistent. This lesion was biopsied and graded as malignant astrocytoma. Malignant astrocytomas represent a middle grade of glioma, less malignant than glioblastoma multiforme (see Case 1), and more aggressive than benign astrocytomas (see Cases 39 and 46). These lesions might be expected to show non-specific uptake on isotope studies. Vessel displacement and mild tumour vessels would be evident on angiography. MRI would fail to show the calcification (an important drawback) but should show the lesion; gadolinium enhancement might also demonstrate the interface between tumour and surrounding oedema.

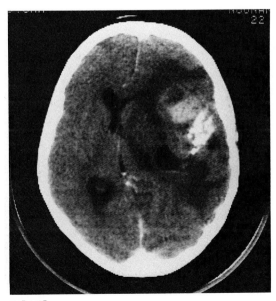

C [+C]

Case 31

Male, aged 24 years.
Slowly progressive left-sided weakness for 6 years.

Q: What possible diagnoses are suggested by the
    arteriogram on this patient?

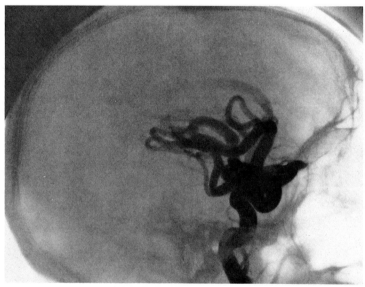

A

Case 31   Arteriovenous malformation (AVM)

An arteriogram is a complete study of sequential films over several seconds and in at least two projections. A single arteriogram film taken in isolation can be very deceptive, as information essential for a complete diagnosis may only be visible on other films from the same series. This case demonstrates that point. The lateral arteriogram film shows enlargement and tortuosity of the internal carotid artery and branches of the middle cerebral artery. This appearance could be due to a tumour, but there is little to suggest an associated mass effect. Dilated tortuous arteries may be seen supplying AVMs but there is no evidence of the early venous filling seen in that condition. However, image B below is the next film in the arteriographic sequence: it was taken about half a second after image A. This clearly shows the knot of small vessels at the site of the fistula and large draining veins leading away from the lesion to their points of drainage in the superior sagittal sinus. Such a rapid transit of blood to the veins may be seen in malignant tumours, however, when present to this degree it is more characteristic of arteriovenous fistulae. These lesions are more fully described in Case 9.

A fistula between a single artery and vein may be seen in the cavernous sinus, where trauma or an aneurysm has allowed the carotid siphon to communicate directly with the sinus in which it lies. MRI will show most AVMs directly since the rapidly moving blood produces signal defects on certain pulse sequences; haemosiderin from previous haemorrhage may also be demonstrated.

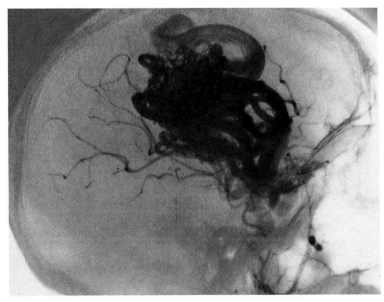

B

Case 32

Female, aged 81 years.
Progressive weakness of left side of body for 6 weeks.
Increasing headaches, moderate papilloedema.

Q: This image was obtained. What important
features are present?

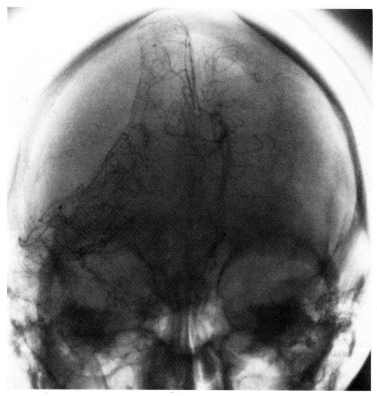

A

Case 32   Chronic subdural haematoma

Image A is a frontal projection of a right carotid arteriogram in the late arterial phase. The film has not been subtracted since the bony structures are still visible, but the image is a negative copy of the original. This shows the vessels black as on a subtracted film but the bone detail is retained. The midline arteries in the anterior cerebral artery complex are displaced to the left, indicating a mass effect on the right side. This has resulted from a lens-shaped collection lying outside the right cerebral hemisphere and causing a curved inward displacement of the small arteries of the cerebral convexity. Such an appearance could conceivably be produced by an extra-axial tumour such as a meningioma but there is no tumour circulation. A more likely cause is a haematoma in the extradural or subdural space. Extradural haematomas do develop this characteristic lens shape but are only found in patients with very recent head injury, i.e., within 48 hours. The long story in this patient indicates that the process has been more gradual and is almost certainly a chronic subdural haematoma. These appearances confirm how the encapsulated haematoma can develop these curved margins as fluid pressure rises within it (see Case 7). Its location has produced local pressure on the motor cortex resulting in hemiparesis, and its space-occupying characteristics account for the history of headache and papilloedema. Where CT is available angiography is no longer necessary to make this diagnosis.

Image B below shows the CT scan of a patient with a subdural haematoma in the isodense phase. The collection itself is not visible as it is the same density as brain, but its presence can be inferred from the compression of the left lateral ventricle. Scans at a lower level showed midline shift. The margin of such a lesion may show enhancement.

Image C shows an isodense haematoma that has developed layers of different density due to sedimentation of its solid and liquid components.

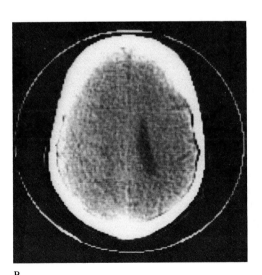

B

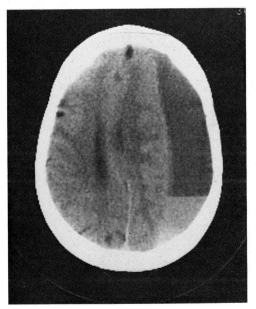

C

Case 33

Male, aged 31 years.
Slowly progressive right hemiparesis for 3 years.

Q: This enhanced CT scan was obtained. What important anatomical structure is displaced and compressed?

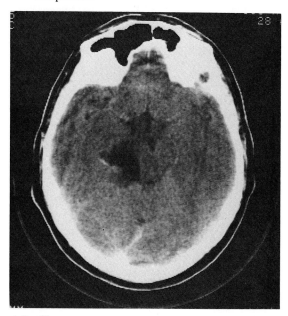

A [+C]

Case 34

Male, aged 5 years.
Six-month history of generalized weakness of limbs, mostly on the right.
Some intellectual loss and scattered neurological deficits.

Q: This T2-weighted spin-echo sequence was obtained. Can you detect any abnormality?

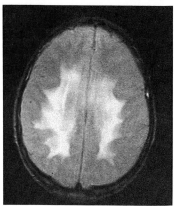

Case 33   Epidermoid (cholesteatoma or 'pearly' tumour)

There is a low-density lesion lying to the left of the upper brainstem. This is causing compression and displacement of the left cerebral peduncle which lies just medial to it (hence the hemiparesis). Other slices showed the lesion extending through the tentorial opening down to the level of the cerebello-pontine angle. The small area of enhancement along its lateral margin was judged to be a displaced, but otherwise normal vascular structure. The density of this lesion is close to that of CSF in the interpeduncular system. The diagnostic possibilities include astrocytoma and arachnoid cysts. This lesion is in fact an epidermoid tumour, and is discussed further in Case 4. They may occur anywhere in the brain or vault but are usually laterally placed, unlike dermoids which tend to be in the midline. Because they contain keratin rather than ordinary fat, they may not show the characteristic low density of fat on CT scans. MRI scans, on the other hand, may show their lipid nature by high signal on both T1- and T2-weighted sequences. Such an appearance is shown on image B (T1-weighted coronal) where a high-signal lesion lies to the left of the brainstem within the apex of the petrous bone.

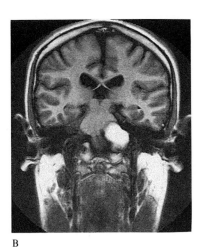

B

Case 34   Adrenoleucodystrophy

The posterior part of the white matter shows high signal areas bilaterally due to demyelination. The slice has been taken through the upper ventricles.

The pattern of symmetrical high signal in the white matter posteriorly is very suggestive of adrenoleuco-dystrophy. This is one of a group of uncommon demyelinating conditions found in patients of all ages: from Alexander's disease in infants, to metachromatic leucodystrophy in adults. This case is typical of a type associated with adrenal dysfunction that is found in young boys. CT shows symmetrical low-density areas in the occipital white matter. The disease is relentlessly progressive and severe brain atrophy results.

Case 35

Male, aged 34 years.
Three-week history of right-sided weakness.
Known case of AIDS.

Q: The CT scans shown below were obtained. What
lesions are shown, and what is the relevence of the
patient's immune status?

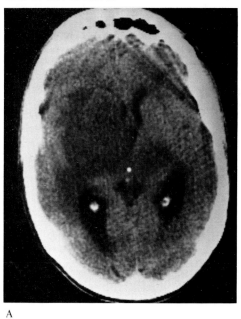

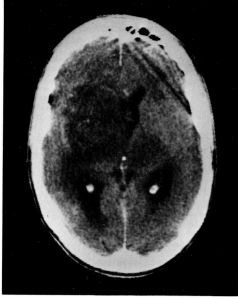

A   B [+C]

Case 36

Male, aged 63 years.
Left hemiparesis for 7 months.

Q: This plain CT scan was obtained. There was no
change after enhancement. What is your
diagnosis?

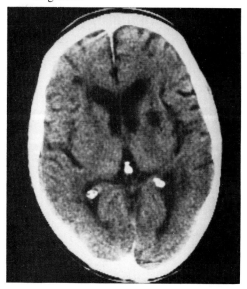

Case 35   Cerebral toxoplasmosis due to AIDS

Image A is a plain CT scan and shows a fairly well-defined low-density area deep in the left hemisphere with compression and displacement of ventricles to the right. A further lesion is present in the right thalamus. Following enhancement there is some increased density along the lateral margin of the larger lesion. These appearances are not specific. The pattern does not suggest infarction, and metastases could be expected to show more enhancement. The presence of a second lesion makes the diagnosis of an astrocytoma highly unlikely; other benign masses such as epidermoids would also have to be considered.

The documentation of this patient's Acquired Immune Deficiency Syndrome provides the essential clue to the cause of the lesion. Neurological symptoms are common in AIDS patients (around 40 per cent), and intracerebral complications include lymphoma and opportunistic infections such as cryptococcal meningitis, toxoplasmosis, progressive multifocal leucoencephalopathy and viral meningitis/encephalitis. Cerebral toxoplasmosis can present in a variety of forms including intracerebral masses (such as this), or meningeal/ependymal reactions. The masses may be of decreased or of raised density and present varying degrees of enhancement, some showing the features of abscesses. A significant proportion of AIDS patients show diffuse cerebral atrophy, possibly due to a low-grade cerebral infection with HIV.

Case 36   Lacunar infarct

The scan shows mild generalized atrophy in keeping with the patient's age. A well-defined low-density area is present in the right anterior internal capsule. A further smaller lesion is seen lateral to the tip of the left frontal horn. The former lesion has a density close to that of CSF and could be cystic. Therefore a cystic tumour is a possibility in this site. However, previous infarcts or small haemorrhages in this region can leave a well-defined area of brain softening which may or may not be cystic. The story revealed that the onset of symptoms had been sudden and the patient's overall status had remained unchanged over the 7 months.

The diagnosis is clearly that of a residual defect from a haemorrhage or infarction. The presence of a second lesion makes the latter diagnosis more probable. Infarcts of this type are called 'lacunes' and are caused by occlusion of a small vessel supplying the basal nuclear area, usually one of the lenticulostriate branches of the middle cerebral artery (*see* Case 22 and *Figure 55*). Despite its small size, an infarct in the internal capsule, corona radiata or cerebral peduncle can produce considerable neurological deficit as major nerve pathways pass through these areas from the cortex.

Speech disorders

General considerations

Speech is a highly complex intellectual and physical attainment and is heavily dependent on the proper functioning of the auditory, visual, motor and memory systems. Disorders of speech are divided into those affecting the comprehension, formulation and expression of words (dysphasia or aphasia), and those where words can be formulated but not pronounced because of a physical impediment such as a cranial nerve palsy (dysarthria).

The 'speech area' of the brain is located adjacent to the Sylvian fissure in the dominant hemisphere. In right-handers this is in the left hemisphere. In left-handed persons the left hemisphere is also usually the seat of the speech area, but right-hemisphere lesions may produce some dysphasia in these patients. The terms 'dysphasia' and 'aphasia' are often used synonymously, but 'aphasia' should be reserved for total loss of speech functions. The receptive speech area (Wernicke) is posteriorly placed and the expressive speech area (Broca) is more anteriorly placed. Thus, dysphasia may be receptive (sensory), expressive (motor) or mixed, depending on the site of the lesion. Vascular, inflammatory, neoplastic and other processes may involve the speech area directly or by distortion of the area from a remote location. Very brief attacks of dysphasia may be encountered in migraine or in transient ischaemic attacks. These symptoms are always worthy of further investigation (in suitably fit patients). Plain skull films and a chest radiograph may provide valuable related evidence of raised intracranial pressure or neoplastic lung lesions for example. CT will usually reveal the causative pathology, but angiography may be needed for further assessment where a vascular cause seems likely. MRI will show these lesions, but apart from evaluation of white matter disease probably has little real advantage over CT in the assessment of aphasia.

Dysarthria can be caused by some lesions in the cerebral hemispheres. Pseudobulbar palsy is due to bilateral corticobulbar upper motor neurone lesions and produces dysarthria. Causes include infarction and motor neurone disease. Lesions in the cerebellum and extrapyramidal system may also produce dysarthria. The motor nuclei in the brainstem (VII, IX, X, XI, XII) are involved in the production of speech, and any lesion in the stem affecting their nuclei or lesions of the nerves or their respective muscles can produce a speech defect. Detailed neurological examination is required to distinguish focal lesions from generalized disorders and imaging techniques will be indicated where the former are suspected. Detailed plain films, perhaps with tomography, may be very helpful when a specific cranial nerve appears to be involved. Occasionally, doubtful bony involvement may have to be confirmed with isotope studies. High-resolution CT scanning with enhancement will reveal many of the space-occupying lesions but small brainstem or cranial nerve lesions would be better demonstrated with MRI. Intrathecally enhanced CT can provide exquisite delineation of the intracranial portions of these nerves. Vertebral angiography has limited value in these cases.

Cases presenting with dysphasia or dysarthria are discussed on the following pages. Other lesions capable of causing these symptoms are found elsewhere under other clinical presentations.

Infarction
Primary brain tumours
Metastases
Post-traumatic atrophy
Glomus jugulare tumour
Choroid plexus papilloma
Cerebral abscess (Case 17)
Encephalitis (Case 15)
Cerebral granuloma (Case 12)
Transient ischaemic attack (Case 48)
Brainstem lesions (Cases 78 and 85)
Arteritis (Case 27)

Case 37

Male, aged 55 years.
Onset of moderate dysphasia 2 weeks ago. Now improving.

Q: The CT scan in image A was obtained together with a left carotid arteriogram. Why was the arteriogram obtained, and what abnormality is present?

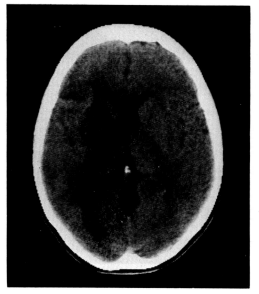

A

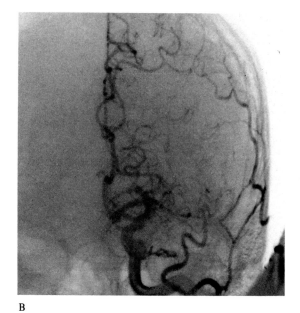

B

Case 37   Occlusion of middle cerebral artery

The CT scan shows only vague low density in the left temporal area, and in view of the history it was considered essential to exclude significant arterial disease in this otherwise fit patient. The arteriogram film is an AP projection and shows a normal appearance in the territory of the anterior cerebral artery. The left middle cerebral artery territory is not perfused however (the vessels filling laterally are branches of the external carotid artery—occipital and superficial temporal arteries). This is most probably due to an embolus arising from atheroma in the internal carotid artery, or the heart valves.

The appearance of the carotid arteriogram in lateral projection is shown below (C and D). Image C confirms the good filling of the anterior cerebral vessels and the largely avascular area in the distribution of the middle cerebral branches. The posterior cerebral artery is filled and passes posteriorly in its usual position. Image D, taken 3 seconds later, shows delayed filling of the middle cerebral branches. This has occurred retrogradely via collateral vessels out in the cortex. It is this substitute circulation which has helped prevent a major infarction, permitted significant clinical recovery for the patient, and accounted for minimal changes on CT. Further discussion on infarction is given in Case 22. Other examples of middle cerebral infarcts are described in Cases 29 and 36.

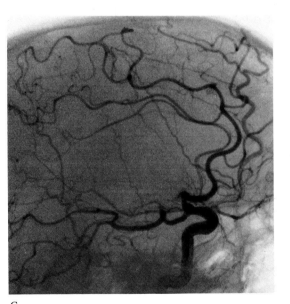

C

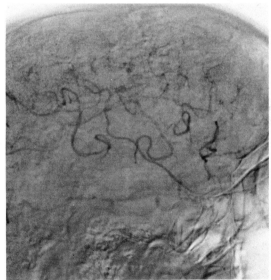

D

Case 38

Female, aged 19 years.
One-year history of speech difficulty with weakness of
the left shoulder. Found to have palsies of VIIth, IXth
and XIth cranial nerves on the left.

Q: This plain-film study and MRI scan were
    obtained. In what anatomical plane have they
    been taken, and what abnormalities are present?

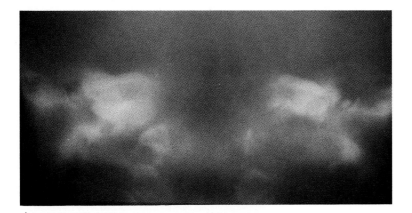

A

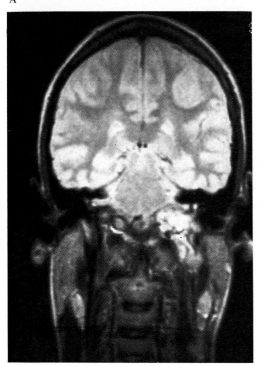

B

Case 38   Glomus jugulare tumour

Image A is a conventional tomograph in the coronal plane. It has been taken through the petrous bone at the level of the middle ear and shows the ossicles clearly on both sides. On the inferior aspect of the right petrous bone, various grooves and channels can be seen. These are mostly due to the normal jugular fossa. On the left side this area is grossly enlarged and expanded. The margins of the expansion are smooth, suggesting a benign process rather than the destruction seen in metastatic disease. These changes suggest a tumour in the jugular fossa, most likely a 'glomus jugulare'. The MRI scan has also been obtained in the coronal plane at approximately the same level (note the 'frontal' view of C2 and the odontoid peg), and is a T2-weighted spin-echo sequence. In the centre of the image a roughly diamond-shaped area of moderately low signal is due to the brainstem with cerebellar peduncles on either side. These are contained within an area of higher signal also diamond-shaped. On the right side this shows a narrow 'tongue' of high signal extending to the right into an area of no signal. This high-signal area represents CSF in the normal cerebello-pontine angle extending into the internal auditory canal. On the left this appearance is distorted by a large high-signal mass below it and extending downwards into the neck. Within this area some serpiginous structures of low signal are seen due to dilated tortuous blood vessels. These changes are also consistent with a tumour in the jugular fossa and shows its extension into the neck.

Tumours of the glomus jugulare are uncommon benign lesions originating in chemoreceptor cells lying in the wall of the jugular vein where it passes through the petrous bone (jugular bulb). The vein is occluded by the lesion and there is pressure on the cranial nerves which emerge through the jugular foramen (IXth, Xth, XIth). In this case the speech difficulty was due to dysarthria from involvement of the IXth nerve. Shoulder weakness was due to involvement of the accessory nerve (XIth). These lesions are slow-growing but difficult to treat as they are highly vascular. A similar tumour occurs at the bifurcation of the common carotid artery.

The enhanced CT scan on this patient is shown below (image C). This confirms the bony erosion of the petrous bone and enhancement can be seen extending into the lower part of the posterior fossa on the left. Angiography confirmed the presence of a vascular mass supplied mostly from posterior branches of the external carotid artery (image D).

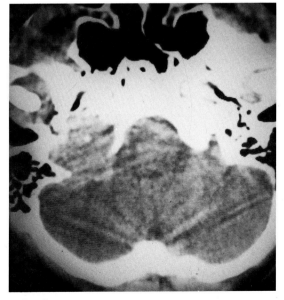

C [+C]

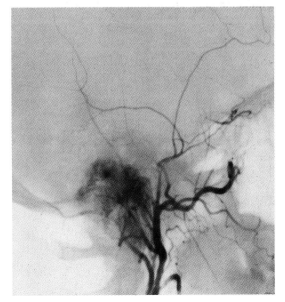

D

Case 39

Female, aged 38 years.
Fifteen-month history of progressive dysphasia.

i   Postinfective calcification.
ii Physiological calcification in basal ganglia.
iii Calcified tumour.
iv AVM.

Q: Which of these diagnoses would you consider on these CT appearances? There was no change after contrast enhancement:

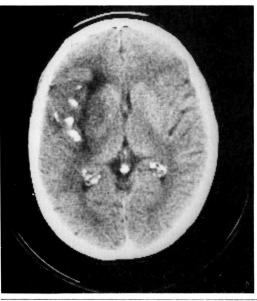

Case 40

Male, aged 41 years.
Mild dysphasia since head injury (RTA) 3 years previously.

Q: What post-traumatic intracerebral process may have resulted in this lesion?

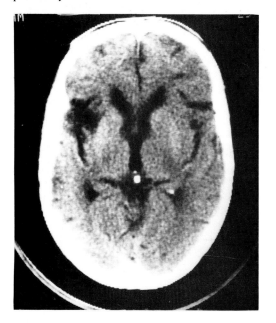

Case 39   Calcified astrocytoma

The CT scan shows irregular calcification just lateral to the left Sylvian fissure and lying therefore within the temporal lobe. This is associated with an ill-defined low-density area in the Sylvian fissure and extending anteriorly and posteriorly from it. There is a slight mass effect with posterior displacement of the left choroid plexus in the trigone, minor midline shift to the right and minimal compression of the left frontal horn.

Postinfective calcification is a late result of that pathology and would be expected to show associated atrophy rather than mass effect. The basal ganglia lie medial to the Sylvian fissure, therefore this cannot be calcification within those structures. AVMs show prominent enhancement (*see* Case 9) which this case did not.

The combination of calcification and low-density area with mass effect is highly suggestive of a calcified tumour. This is most likely to be an oligo-dendroglioma (Case 8) or astrocytoma. The former have a predilection for the frontal lobes. Calcification may be seen within gliomas of all grades (*see* Case 30), but when enhancement is absent a low-grade tumour is likely.

Case 40   Post-traumatic scarring

This CT scan shows an area of focal atrophy around the anterior part of the left Sylvian fissure. The fissure is widened and there is slight displacement of midline structures towards this side, indicating loss of volume in this hemisphere. A previous head injury may have produced a focal haemorrhage, contusion or even infarction. Even when due to trauma, infarction tends to follow a vascular pattern which is not present in this case. Extracerebral collections without intracerebral lesions do not usually produce focal damage of this kind. A CT scan at the time of injury had shown an area of contusion with oedema and small foci of haemorrhage in this area. The lesion was very close to the speech area and the patient exhibited marked dysphasia at the time of the injury. Recovery from this dysphasia had been incomplete.

Case 41

Female aged 47.
Receptive dysphasia for 5 weeks.

Q: Can you make a definitive diagnosis from the
appearances shown on this patient's CT scan?

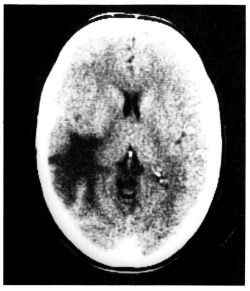

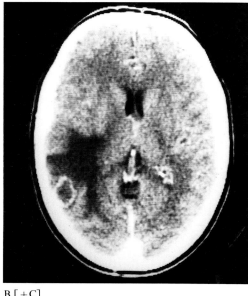

A

B [+C]

Case 42

Male aged 8 years.
Eight-month history of dysphasia and headaches.

Q: This enhanced CT scan shows a gross
abnormality. How does this scan explain the
patient's symptoms?

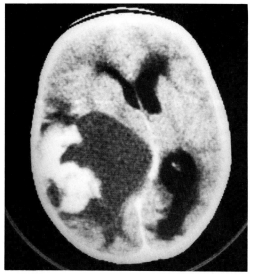

[+C]

Case 41   Metastatic deposit

These CT scans show a ring-like area of enhancement within a zone of oedema located in the posterior temporal and parietal regions of the left hemisphere. There were no other lesions and consequently a wide range of differential diagnoses has to be considered. Abscess, glioma, granuloma or solitary metastatic deposit all have to be considered. The extensive oedema lies mostly anterior to the lesion and extends into the receptive speech area. A close examination of the patient revealed an early carcinoma of the breast, thereby avoiding the biopsy which is so often required to finalize the diagnosis in a single lesion with this appearance.

Contrast enhancement should be given if metastatic disease is suspected; also, the absence of enhancement effectively excludes this diagnosis in a mass lesion within the brain. Prominent oedema is a common feature of metastatic deposits but calcification is rarely seen.

Case 42   Choroid plexus papilloma

The lesion is composed of an enhancing area laterally in the temporal lobe with a low-density area deep to it. This latter structure is not as low in density as CSF and may be a cystic part of the enhancing mass. It could, however, be a portion of the lateral ventricle which has become isolated by the local distortion and contains proteinaceous CSF. The location of this lesion is very close to the speech areas, thereby accounting for the dysphasia. The mass itself could produce headache, but there is also moderate hydrocephalus shown by the ventricular dilatation and oedematous areas around the frontal horns.

This tumour is uncommon and does not usually grow to this size. It arises within the ventricle from the choroid plexus and causes obstruction of the ventricular pathways. It may also stimulate the production of excessive amounts of CSF. Both these effects frequently result in hydrocephalus. Prominent enhancement is usually evident and some tumours may seed through the CSF spaces to other locations.

Seizures

General considerations

This chapter deals with a variety of attacks with which patients may present. Most of these are epileptic seizures or variants of that entity, but other causes of brief loss or alteration of consciousness are also discussed.

Epileptic seizures result from abnormal synchronous electrical activity within the brain. Most cases are idiopathic in origin. Many different patterns of epileptic seizures are recognized, including grand mal, petit mal, temporal lobe, focal, motor, etc. The most important differentiation is between generalized or partial attacks. These various types can usually be differentiated by the history and eyewitness accounts.

The need to investigate a patient with seizures is dependent on a number of factors. The patient's age is very important. Most cases of idiopathic epilepsy commence in childhood and in the presence of a typical story (which may involve a family history); imaging investigations are rarely required. It is also common to encounter fairly typical epileptic-type attacks in feverish children without a previous history (febrile convulsions). These invariably pass with recovery of the precipitating illness. Further investigation is therefore rarely indicated. Where the fit follows a story of trauma, or is focal and associated with neurological deficits, then investigation by diagnostic imaging is indicated.

In older patients the duration of the story is of vital importance. A further seizure of the usual pattern in a patient with a history of seizures dating back to childhood is not a cause for concern. A change in seizure pattern or loss in seizure control are reasonable grounds for suspicion. In adults without a history of previous seizures, a first attack (late-onset epilepsy) is usually a signal for detailed investigation, as there may be an underlying focal lesion such as a tumour or infarct. This is particularly true in seizures which suggest a focal origin such as temporal lobe epilepsy, or fits starting in one limb and then becoming more generalized. Seizures associated with neurological deficit or following trauma merit further investigation. EEG evaluation is useful in the diagnosis and management of seizures but its value in predicting which patients will merit investigation by imaging techniques is limited (in our experience).

It is clear, therefore, that a detailed history and physical examination should provide a sound basis on which a decision about further investigation can be based. Simple physical details such as adenoma sebaceum, port-wine stain or asymmetry of the head or limbs may point to a specific underlying cause (see Cases 51, 53 and 54).

In those cases outlined above, and where imaging is being embarked upon, plain films may show a variety of important features including intracranial calcification, raised intracranial pressure, cranial hemiatrophy, etc. Isotope studies may be helpful where CT is not available, but CT is the principal diagnostic technique. Angiography is usually only indicated where CT indicates a possible underlying vascular cause such as infarction or an AVM. MRI is certainly capable of demonstrating most of the causative lesions, but its advantages, if any, over the more readily available CT in investigations of this condition have yet to be established. In infants, cranial ultrasound may reveal underlying intracerebral haematoma, subdural collection or hydrocephalus.

Apart from 'fits', patients may present with other attacks of altered consciousness due to syncope, migraine, thromboembolic disease, hypoglycaemia, etc. The underlying nature of these is usually obvious from the history. Thromboembolic events, usually known as 'transient ischaemic attacks' (TIAs), are particularly important as they may herald a complete stroke. These TIAs are usually encountered in older patients and are characterized by transient weakness, dysphasia or blindness. Unconsciousness is unusual except where the brainstem is involved. Further investigation is warranted to confirm the diagnosis in cases where some doubt exists, and for those in whom surgical treatment of the underlying vascular disease is a practical proposition. There are a number of non-invasive techniques which can detect the presence of a vascular cause, but where definitive studies are required for surgical decisions or where intracranial atheroma needs to be excluded, then arteriography will be required. Intravenous digital subtraction can provide a useful assessment of the carotid vessels in the neck. CT can be very helpful as a few patients with classic TIAs turn out to have a cerebral tumour. It is important to note that late-onset focal epilepsy can sometimes be mistaken for TIAs.

Lesions which may produce seizures and have imaging manifestations are listed below. A case of transient ischaemic attacks is also described in the ensuing cases.

Intracranial cysts
Cerebral infarction
AVM
Cerebral haemorrhage
Old cerebral trauma
Metastatic deposit
Primary cerebral tumours
Developmental lesions
   Sturge–Weber Syndrome
   Tuberous sclerosis
   Neurofibromatosis (Case 10)
Hydrocephalus (Case 63)
Extradural haematoma (Case 66)
Subdural haematoma (Case 65)
Encephalitis (Case 15)
Meningitis/abscess (Case 17)
Cerebral granulomas (Case 12)
Leucodystrophy (Case 34)

Case 43

Male, aged 53 years.
Generalized epileptic convulsions for 8 weeks.

Q: What possible diagnoses would you consider for
    the appearances on these images?

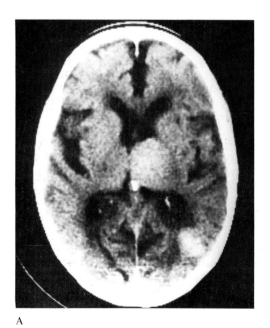

A

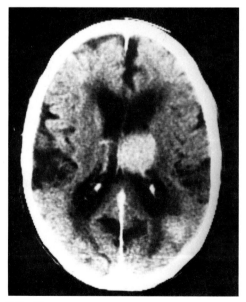

B [+C]

Case 43   Metastatic disease

These CT scan images show two areas of raised density in the right hemisphere. After enhancement, these show only a mild increase in density. Multiple masses such as these may be due to meningiomas, neuromas, abscesses, granulomas, metastases, or lymphoma. The larger of these lesions is in the thalamus, a most unusual site for a meningioma which would also show more enhancement than this. Neuromas are usually found along the courses of cranial nerves. Abscesses show ring-shaped enhancement. Granulomas show a variety of appearances and could look like this. Lymphoma also shows high-density lesions on the plain scans but is characterized by intense enhancement (see Case 93).

Metastatic disease is the commonest cause of multiple masses in the brain and should be strongly suspected in a patient with these appearances. Most metastases are isodense, or of lower density than brain on plain scans and show irregular areas of enhancement (see Case 3). Metastases of high density

are sometimes seen from malignant melanoma or certain bowel tumours. The high density may be due to haemorrhage or additionally (in the case of melanoma) melanin. This patient had a mucinous carcinoma of the colon removed 2 years previously; a biopsy confirmed that these were metastases from that primary.

Metastatic deposits may also present as a cause of hydrocephalus. A particularly difficult diagnostic problem may be encountered in patients with deposits or sheets of metastatic cells along the meninges or arachnoid space. Such patients have unusual combinations of cranial nerve signs and the CT may be unremarkable. In some cases, however, the process may be evident as vague areas of enhancement in the basal cisterns. Such a case is shown below in images C and D. Image C shows an enhancing lesion in the right cerebello-pontine angle and in the Sylvian fissure areas. Image D shows diffuse uptake along the tentorium and in both Sylvian fissures.

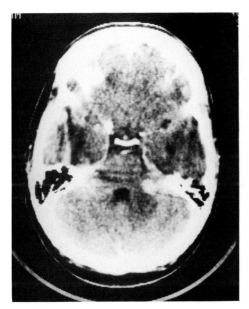

C [+C]

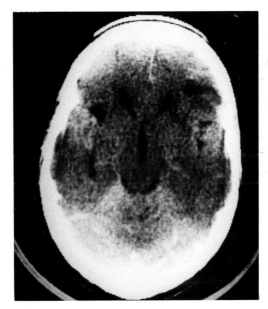

D [+C]

Case 44

Female, aged 39 years.
Generalized seizures since the age of 8 years.
Recently more frequent with increasing headaches.

Q: What does this plain film show (A)? How does
    this relate to the changes on this patient's CT scan
    (B)?

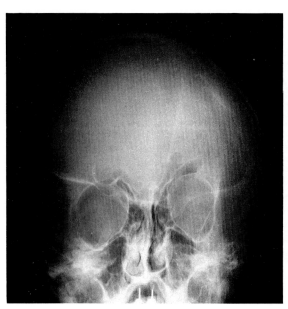

A

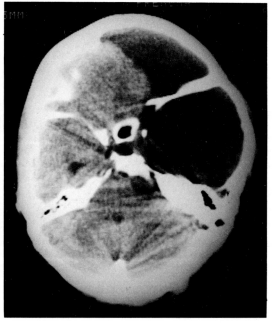

B

Case 44   Arachnoid cyst

The plain film shows considerable expansion of the right anterior cranial fossa and there is associated downward displacement of the right orbit and frontal sinus. The right hemicranium is also enlarged compared with the left. These features suggest a longstanding mass effect in these areas. Similar findings are also present on the CT scan. The right side of the vault is bigger than the left and there is specific enlargement of the right middle and anterior cranial fossae by a large well-defined area of low density. This cystic area must have been present for many years to have produced these changes in the modelling of the skull. The appearances are those of a giant arachnoid cyst.

Cysts in the arachnoid space are quite a common finding in the cranial cavity. Most communicate with the arachnoid space and this can be demonstrated with intrathecal contrast medium when doubt about the diagnosis exists. The most frequent sites for these lesions are the Sylvian fissures or suprasellar cisterns. Their density is that of CSF. They may also be found in the posterior fossa. In many instances small cysts are an incidental finding and asymptomatic. Larger cysts cause focal pressure effects as in this case and patients may benefit from having the cyst shunted. Cysts of the size found in this patient are unusual. A more typical size and appearance of arachnoid cyst is shown in image C below. Here the well-defined low-density area is within the left Sylvian fissure, which has been expanded by the cyst displacing the adjacent frontal and temporal lobes. There is also some bony expansion and mass effect. This patient presented with mild right-sided weakness.

These cysts may also be shown on MRI scanning but as yet there is little evidence to suggest that this technique has a significant contribution to make to the diagnosis. Angiography may show non-specific displacement of vessels adjacent to the larger cysts. The principal differential diagnoses of these lesions are porencephalic cysts (*see* Case 45) and cystic tumours (*see* Case 46).

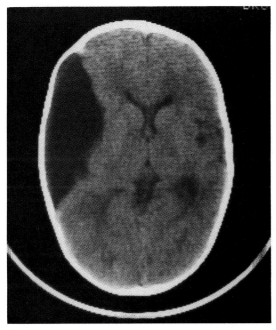

C

Case 45

Male, aged 17 years.
Focal seizures since brain surgery, 3 years previously.

Q: These CT appearances are consistent with which
    diagnosis? (There was no change after contrast
    enhancement.)

    i   Cystic glioma.
    ii Arachnoid cyst.
    iii Porencephalic cyst.

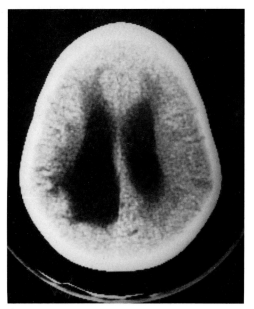

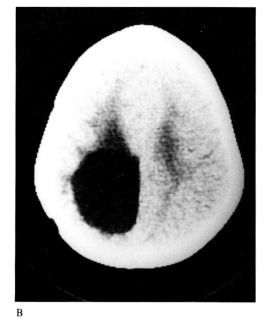

A   B

Case 45   Porencephalic cyst

These unenhanced CT scans show a well-defined low-density area in the upper left hemisphere. Its density is the same as that of the CSF in the ventricles. On image A it can be seen that there is no interface between this 'cyst' and the adjacent ventricle, in fact these two structures are in continuity. Irregularity of the vault in the left parietal area is due to the previous surgery. The appearances are consistent with a diagnosis of porencephalic cyst.

A porencephalic cyst is a focal dilatation of the ventricular system into a localized area of atrophic brain. In the majority of cases a lateral ventricle is involved. Loss of brain substance from trauma, infarction, surgery, etc. may be the cause of this appearance. The damaged area of parenchyma shrinks, dragging the ventricle towards it, to take up the vacant space. The communication between the dilated area and its parent ventricle may be difficult to establish. Their continuity can be confirmed by opacification of the ventricles with contrast medium. In some, the communication is intermittent and the cystic area enlarges producing a mass effect. These lesions may produce seizures, weakness, sensory loss, dysphasia, etc., depending on their location. Some of these symptoms may be the result of the focal damage rather than the cyst.

Other cysts can show a superficial resemblance to this condition. Cystic tumours, notably gliomas, would not show a communication with the ventricle (*see* Case 46). Enhancement may also be present in such tumours. Arachnoid cysts do not communicate with the ventricle (*see* Case 44) and occur in specific sites such as the Sylvian fissure. Epidermoid cysts tend to be somewhat denser than this and are mostly seen along the base (*see* Case 33).

Case 46

Male, aged 44 years.
Grand mal seizures for 3½ months.

Q: This definitive study was obtained. What is your
    diagnosis? There was no change after contrast
    enhancement.

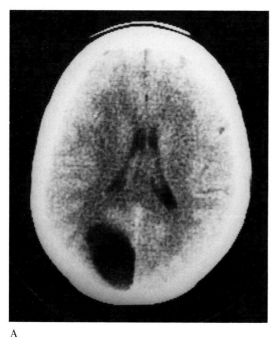

A

Case 46   Cystic astrocytoma

This CT scan shows a well-defined low-density area in the left occipital area that is producing some forward displacement of the posterior part of the left lateral ventricle. The density of the lesion is close to that of CSF but there was nothing to suggest that it communicated with the ventricle as a porencephalic cyst would do (*see* Case 45). Arachnoid cysts are unusual in this site (*see* Case 44). Cysts following haemorrhage are not usually space-taking but rather 'atrophic' (*see* Case 76). This lesion was biopsied and found to be a cystic astrocytoma.

These tumours are at the lower end of the scale of malignancy in gliomas (*see* Case 1). They may show some enhancement in the margin of the cyst, but this is not usually a striking feature. Some of these lesions appear cystic on CT but are found to be solid at operation; histology, however, shows myriads of tiny cysts within an otherwise solid lesion, accounting for the low-density values. Such a case is shown below (image B). Low-grade astrocytomas may also present as ill-defined low-density lesions (non-cystic), or partly calcified lesions with little or no enhancement (*see also* Cases 39 and 71). Some lesions can become more malignant with time.

A lesion in this situation might reasonably be expected to produce a visual field defect, and this sign was present. Seizures are produced by local irritation of the cortex and may manifest as a partial or generalized attack.

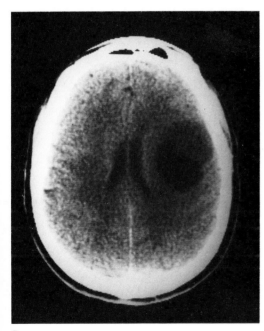

B

Case 47

Female, aged 25 years.
Three-day history of generalized convulsions.
Longstanding mitral valve disease.

Q: A CT scan showed an area of infarction in the left occipital lobe with a bizarre pattern of enhancement. This arteriogram film was subsequently obtained. What does it show?

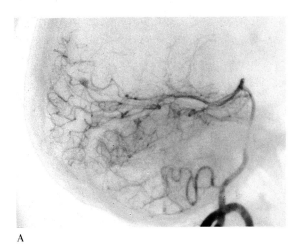

A

Case 48

Male, aged 52 years.
Two-month history of transient visual loss with transient right-sided weakness.

Q: A CT scan was normal. What imaging technique is this? What pathology is shown?

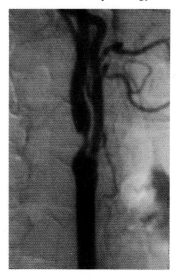

Case 47   Septic infarction with mycotic aneurysm

This is a lateral film from a vertebral arteriogram. A small aneurysm is seen distally in a branch of the posterior cerebral artery. Congenital berry aneurysms

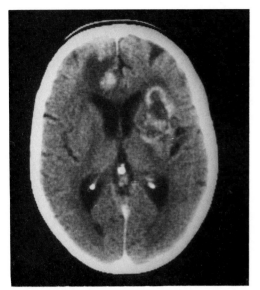

B [+C]

invariably occur around the circle of Willis and an aneurysm this far distally is almost certainly acquired through surgery, trauma or an infected embolus. When emboli occur in bacterial endocarditis, septicaemia or other such situations of systemic infection, they are likely to be infected, and local damage to the occluded vessel may result in mycotic aneurysm. These may present with spontaneous haemorrhage or septic infarction. On CT, septic infarcts appear initially like ordinary infarcts, but have a florid and atypical enhancement (see Case 22 for the usual appearances of infarcts on CT). A further case is shown below (image B) where the CT scan shows a low-density area in the left frontal lobe with a general distribution suggesting anterior cerebral infarction. There is central enhancement. A further lesion is present in the right basal nuclei with marked irregular enhancement. The differential diagnosis is wide and includes metastases, but the infarction pattern is suspicious and this patient was undergoing renal dialysis and had documented septicaemia.

Case 48   Transient cerebral ischaemia due to carotid artery stenosis

This patient's symptoms are consistent with attacks of transient cerebral ischaemia. These TIAs (see p. 143) are characterized by brief, i.e., often less than 1 hour, attacks of ischaemia involving the retina (amaurosis fugax) or any part of the brain, with hemiparesis or other symptoms. These are mostly the result of microemboli of platelets causing brief occlusion of small cerebral vessels. Most of these probably arise from atheromatous plaques in the carotid or vertebral arteries. The commonest site for these atheromatous plaques is at the origin of the internal carotid artery from the common carotid artery. The image shown is part of a left common carotid arteriogram, and shows

narrowing of the origin of the internal carotid by atheroma. The vessel does not need to be tightly stenosed for these emboli to occur. Such lesions may be amenable to carotid endarterectomy with relief of symptoms. There are often no intracerebral changes visible on CT scans unless emboli have produced actual areas of infarction. These areas may be quite small, and single or multiple. They may give rise to true epileptic attacks. Such a focal lesion is shown in Case 75.

The arteriogram film shown has been obtained using digital subtraction.

Case 49

Male, aged 43 years.
Long history of partial seizures.

Q: Plain and enhanced CT scans were obtained. What is your diagnosis, and how might it be further confirmed?

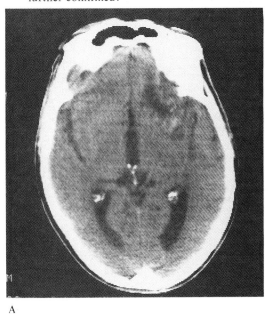

A

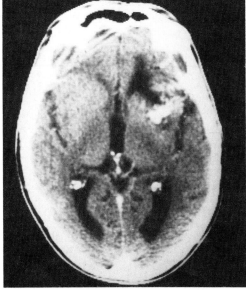

B [+C]

Case 50

Female, aged 36 years.
Three-year history of generalized seizures following surgery and radiotherapy for cerebral tumour.

Q: What possible diagnoses would have to be considered on this clinical information? Does this CT scan confirm any of these possibilities?

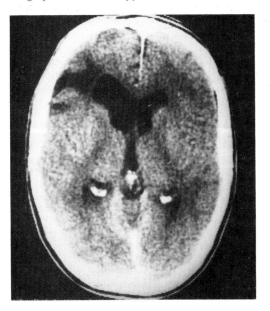

Case 49 Small AVM

The plain scan shows an area of atrophy in the right Sylvian fissure. There are some areas of raised density associated with this. Irregular enhancement is also present in this area on image B. Focal atrophy with enhancement is very suggestive of an AVM (*see* Case 9). These lesions are commonly associated with focal atrophy, perhaps due to ischaemia of the neighbouring tissues or an associated dystrophic change. Seizures are a fairly common presentation for AVMs, and these may be triggered by the presence of the lesion itself or the adjacent atrophy. AVMs are also described in Cases 16 and 31. The lesion can be confirmed and further delineated by angiography and the right carotid arteriogram on this patient shows these features (image C).

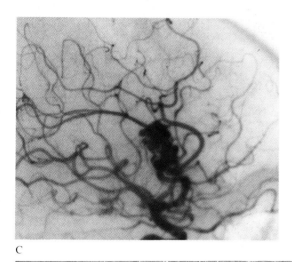

C

Case 50 Brain scarring/softening

Seizures following any brain insult may be a long-term result of the lesion or its sequelae. In the case of surgery for tumour a recurrence would have to be considered. To exclude this possibility, contrast enhancement was given and the appearances were unchanged. A review of previous scans also revealed no change in the appearances over several years. This low-density area is associated with focal dilatation of the lateral ventricle into the area indicating local atrophy. Radiotherapy can produce radiation necrosis, but this is an active process with enhancement and a changing pattern over a period of time. An inactive area of scarring such as this may be the result of local surgery, trauma, haemorrhage or previous radiation therapy. It may be quite impossible to distinguish between these possible causes on the CT appearances, but the clinical history should help.

An area of porencephaly might be mistaken for softening and in fact is produced in a similar way. However, porencephalic cysts result from marked tissue necrosis and they communicate with the ventricle (*see* Case 45).

Case 51

Female, aged 20 years.
Frequent fits since birth with right-sided spastic hemiparesis.

Q: What does this plain film show? What might a CT
      scan be expected to exhibit?

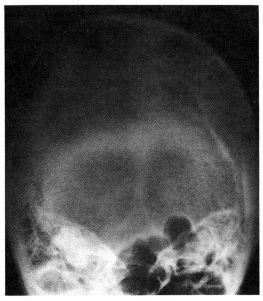

A

Case 52

Male, 4 weeks premature infant. Three generalized
convulsions 6 hours after delivery.

Q: What diagnostic technique is this, and what does
      it show? How might this technique be useful in
      further monitoring of the patient?

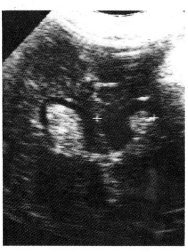

A

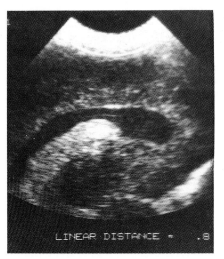

B

Case 51   Hemiatrophy

This plain skull film shows the left side of the vault to be smaller than the right. The vault is also thicker on the left and the frontal sinus on this side is markedly enlarged. There is slight elevation of the left petrous bone. All these features point to a reduction in size of the left cerebral hemisphere. These must be long-standing discrepancies, since infancy in fact, as the skull has not grown to accommodate a normally developing hemisphere. The affected hemisphere is atrophic and this may be a generalized atrophy of that hemisphere or localized to one area. The atrophy may be the result of a vascular insult (probably the commonest cause), or other causes such as trauma, haemorrhage or encephalitis. Image B shows the CT scan of another case where a difficult delivery resulted in vascular trauma. A major infarct in the left middle cerebral territory ensued. The left hemisphere developed less well than the right and is generally smaller with a thickened and less capacious vault on this side. The atrophic area resulting from the middle cerebral infarct can be seen.

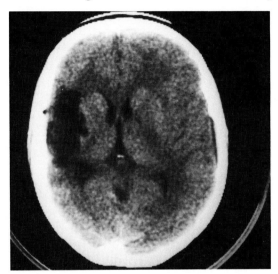

B

Case 52   Intracranial haemorrhage

These are coronal (A) and parasagittal (B) images from an intracranial ultrasound examination. Normal appearances are shown in *Figures 49* and *50*. The images have been obtained through the anterior fontanelle and show mild dilatation of the ventricles. The right lateral ventricle is seen to contain brightly reflective material. This is characteristic of fresh intraventricular haemorrhage, and this ependymal location is frequently seen. Ultrasound can also show haemorrhage into the cerebral substance away from the ventricles.

Acute intracerebral haemorrhage is an important and common condition in premature infants, and may present with convulsions, coma, hemiparesis or signs of intracranial pressure. Ultrasound examination is now well-established in the role of providing front-line diagnosis for such cases. CT or MRI may also demonstrate this type of haemorrhage.

Ultrasound provides a harmless, non-invasive technique for monitoring the progress of these haemorrhages and in demonstrating the development of hydrocephalus, a common result of blood in the ventricular system. A repeat coronal scan on this patient 17 days later showed that the haemorrhage had cleared, but there was now enlargement of the ventricles.

Case 53

Male aged 15 years.
Bizarre form of epileptic seizures.
Mild mental retardation.
Facial rash.

Q: This CT scan was obtained. What is your
    diagnosis?

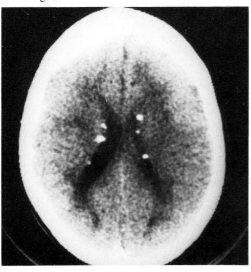

Case 54

Female aged 19 years.
Grand mal epilepsy for many years.
Port-wine stain on cheek.

Q: This plain film shows characteristic changes.
    What is the significance of the facial lesion?

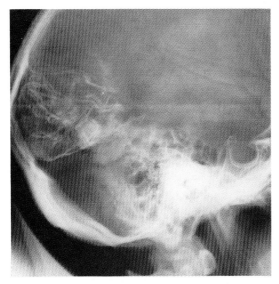

Case 53   Tuberous sclerosis (Bourneville's disease)

This plain CT scan shows 'spots' of calcification in the walls of the ventricular system. There was no change after contrast enhancement. This appearance is practically diagnostic of tuberous sclerosis. This congenital disorder belongs to the group of diseases known as phakomatoses, which are characterized by abnormal development of connective tissue. Afflicted patients may exhibit a variety of manifestations, including hamartomas of the kidneys and these 'tubers' lying in the ependymal linings of the ventricles.

Convulsions are common and a facial rash (adenoma sebaceum) is invariably present. The calcified tubers may be seen on plain skull films in a periventricular distribution. A small proportion of patients develop tumours adjacent to the ventricular wall.

Occasionally it may be helpful to scan the parents of these patients to establish whether a parent has a mild form of the disease. Such a discovery may have an important influence on genetic counselling for the family.

Case 54   Sturge–Weber syndrome

This lateral film shows striking serpiginous calcification in the left occipital area. The calcification runs in curved parallel lines due to its location on the surface of the gyri. This is due to a congenital dystrophic process in the occipital lobe and is typically associated with a capillary haemangioma (purple naevus) on the face. This may be on the opposite side to the occipital lesion. The latter shows the microscopic changes of abnormal vessels but these are not evident on angiography. CT scans will show a rim of calcification outlining the affected atrophic occipital lobe. The adjacent occipital horn of the lateral ventricle is dilated.

Pituitary and parasellar lesions

General considerations

Lesions arising in the pituitary gland or adjacent structures give rise to clinical symptoms, signs and imaging manifestations that form a coherent group. Broadly, the presenting symptoms may be primarily endocrine in type, or exclusively neurological. Both types of presentation are commonly seen together.

Neurological manifestations are many and relate to the many important structures in this region. Obliteration of the suprasellar cisterns, parasellar cisterns, or deformity of the adjacent anterior third ventricle can lead to hydrocephalus. Pressure or distortion of the cranial nerves in this area, i.e., II, III, IV, VI or V, will lead to the appropriate loss of vision, ocular movements or facial sensation. The optic chiasm lies directly above the pituitary fossa and is commonly compressed by lesions in this area. A more detailed account of chiasm involvement is given in the chapter on sensory loss. The sella is surrounded by vascular structures such as the cavernous sinus, the carotid arteries and their major branches. These may in themselves be the source of lesions, or be involved by adjacent pathology. Fractures, surgical changes or tumour invasion may perforate the sellar floor leading to CSF rhinorrhoea.

Pressure from masses within or above the pituitary gland can produce generalized hypopituitarism. Infarction or haemorrhage within the gland commonly result in an acute crisis of hypopituitarism (apoplexy). The spectrum of clinical presentation of raised or lowered pituitary hormone levels is wide and the reader is referred to appropriate texts for such clinical data. Elevated levels of pituitary hormones can be detected or inferred by biochemical tests. Some cases are in response to lesions in other glands but many result from hyperplasia or adenomas in the pituitary. Lesions in the hypothalamus can produce similar effects. Acromegaly and hyperprolactinaemia, however, are very likely to originate in the pituitary. Endocrine disorders need to be thoroughly investigated biochemically before imaging is undertaken.

Patients whose principal presentation is of a neurological disorder, as outlined above, will require plain films and probably CT or MRI scanning. Should the question of a vascular tumour or aneurysm arise from these studies, arteriography may be required for further evaluation. Cranial nerve presentations may indicate pathology in areas other than this, and the occipital regions or posterior fossa may also need to be assessed in patients with appropriate signs. Endocrine manifestations will require a lateral skull film to assess the size and shape of the pituitary fossa. Tomography may be required. CT or MRI scanning are probably not indicated to demonstrate microadenomas unless non-medical management becomes necessary. Larger adenomas can be inferred from the size of the fossa, but surgical management will probably dictate detailed CT or MRI assessment. Angiography may also be needed to demonstrate vascular involvement.

Below are listed some of the commoner causes of pathology in this area. The first seven cases are presented on the ensuing pages.

Pituitary macroadenoma (*also* Case 73)
Pituitary microadenoma
Craniopharyngioma
Empty sella
Optic glioma
Aneurysms
Metastases in skull base
Meningioma
Other cranial nerve neuromas
Hypothalamic glioma
Hydrocephalus (Case 5)
Pituitary infarction

Case 55

Female, aged 40 years.
Four-month history of endocrine disturbance and headaches.

Q: This plain film and the accompanying CT scans were obtained. What differential diagnoses should be considered?

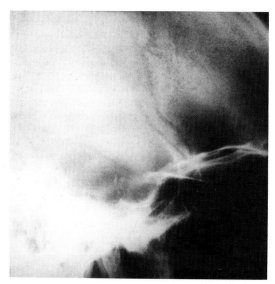

A

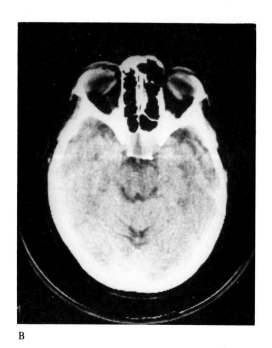

B

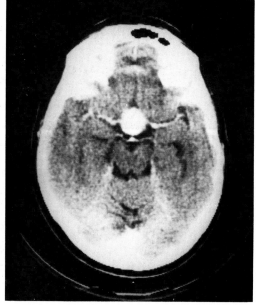

C [+C]

Case 55   Pituitary adenoma

The plain film shows enlargement of the pituitary fossa with thinning and backward tilting of the dorsum sella. Image B is an unenhanced CT scan confirming an enlarged pituitary fossa which contains material of slightly higher density than brain (a dark wedge-shaped artefact from bone overlies the fossa). Image C is taken at a slightly higher level with contrast enhancement and shows the lesion has enhanced and extends into the suprasellar cistern. Scans at a higher level revealed mild hydrocephalus. These appearances are almost certainly due to a pituitary adenoma expanding the fossa and rising up into the suprasellar cistern.

Pituitary adenoma is a common condition and benign adenomas of many types arise within the pituitary gland. Lesions over 10 mm in diameter are usually readily seen on imaging techniques. Many have endocrine manifestations such as in this case. These may be disorders of growth hormone (acromegaly), ACTH production (Cushing's syndrome), hypopituitarism, or hyperprolactinaemia (amenorrhoea and galactorrhoea). Some adenomas have no significant endocrine effects. Any of them can produce headache, compression of optic chiasm or cranial nerves III, IV or VI; or hydrocephalus by obstruction of basal cisterns or upward extension to the foramen of Monro. On CT, contrast enhancement is almost always present. Some adenomas may show cystic change or calcification. Larger lesions may cause displacement of the cavernous portions of the carotid siphons or anterior cerebral arteries on angiography (*see* Case 73). Some also show tumour circulation. The coronal and sagittal capability of MRI may mean that this technique will have a major role in delineating the precise border of these lesions. Such an example is shown in Case 73.

Lesions less than 10 mm are called 'micro-adenomas'. These mostly secrete prolactin but may produce other endocrine syndromes. These small tumours can show focal erosion of the walls of the pituitary that can be seen on tomography of the pituitary fossa. Such a case is shown in D. The location of the defect, however, does not always correspond to the site of the tumour. High-resolution CT scanning, preferably in the coronal plane, can demonstrate focal lesions within the pituitary in such patients, but these are not always at the site of the tumour. In any event, most patients with microadenomas can be managed successfully on bromocriptine and localization is not important.

Some diagnostic difficulty may be enountered in this area, particularly if endocrine manifestations are absent. Well-defined enhancing lesions in this area can also be due to giant aneurysms (*see* Case 57), meningioma (*see* Case 58), craniopharyngioma (*see* Case 56) or optic glioma (*see* Case 59). Cystic changes within pituitary tumours may be confused with an 'empty sella' (*see* Case 61).

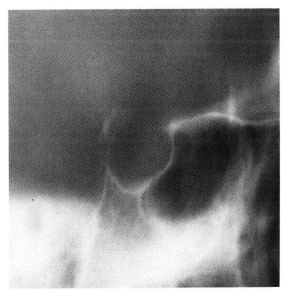

D

Case 56

Female, aged 19 years.
Headache and decreasing vision for 2 years.
Bitemporal hemianopia.

Q: What does this plain skull film show? What
    further tests are indicated?

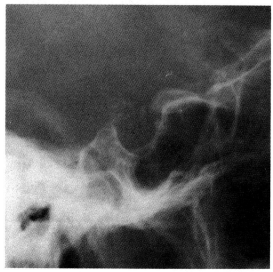

A

Case 56   Craniopharyngioma

This lateral skull film shows two important features. There is some calcification overlying the pituitary fossa; an AP film confirmed this lay directly over the pituitary fossa and not more laterally. The fossa itself is not enlarged but the dorsum sellae is shortened because of erosion superiorly. These features suggest a calcified mass above the sella. Clearly further investigation is warranted. MRI has a major role to play in this region (*see* front cover), but its tendency to 'ignore' calcification may be a problem. Angiography may be needed to exclude an aneurysm or meningioma, but CT would normally be the next imaging technique to further clarify the diagnosis. An unenhanced scan (B) and post-contrast scan (C) on this patient are shown below. Image B is taken through the upper pituitary fossa and shows the clump of calcification. Image C is taken through the third ventricle and shows that the mass extends up to this level occluding the third ventricle and blocking the foramen of Monro to produce hydrocephalus. The lesion is well-defined and of low density, suggesting a cyst. A curve of raised density along its margin is due to enhancement in the wall. The combination of calcification, cystic components and enhancement in a suprasellar lesion is highly suggestive of cranio-pharyngioma.

This benign tumour is of developmental origin and arises in the pituitary fossa or suprasellar area. It usually contains oily brown fluid and can be found at any age but especially in the young. Headaches, optic chiasm compression and hypopituitarism are the principal presenting features. Some of the CT findings described above may be absent.

The differential diagnosis must include meningioma (*see* Case 58), large pituitary tumours (*see* Case 73) and giant aneurysm (*see* Case 57).

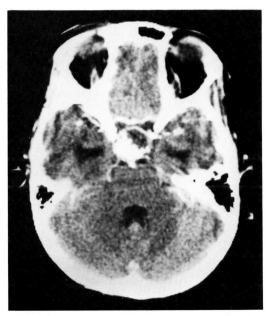

B

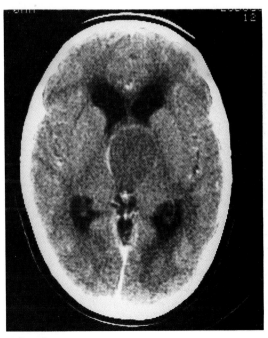

C [+C]

Case 57

Male, aged 62 years.
Headaches for many years.
Recently visual loss and some reduction in sense of smell.

Q: What plain film sign is present?

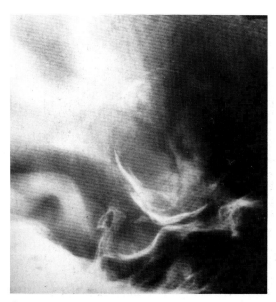

A

Case 57   Parasellar aneurysm

This lateral skull film shows a normal size pituitary fossa, but a ring-shaped area of calcification can be seen just anterior to the fossa. An AP film confirmed that this lay in the midline. Such an appearance could be due to a calcified meningioma or an aneurysm. The latter is more likely as it would be unusual for a meningioma to be completely calcified around its margin. Angiography showed only a mass. Some large aneurysms may not fill on angiography due to the presence of clot (*see* Case 83). At surgery a large aneurysm was found arising from the anterior communicating artery. Pressure on the olfactory cortex and optic chiasm was relieved and the patient's symptoms recovered.

Giant aneurysms most commonly arise from the termination of the internal carotid artery (*see* image B) but may be found at any of the usual sites for aneurysms (*see* Case 13). The symptoms may be headache, hydrocephalus or local pressure effects.

CT appearances will depend on the degree of calcification and/or thrombosis present. A dense lesion with enhancement is shown in image C below, from another patient. Some aneurysms may arise from the medial aspect of the siphon and present within the fossa. This possibility should be considered in any pituitary mass that shows marked enhancement.

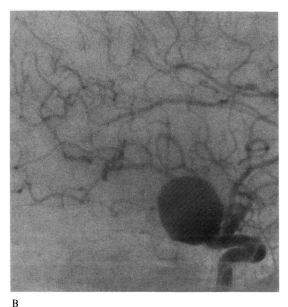

B

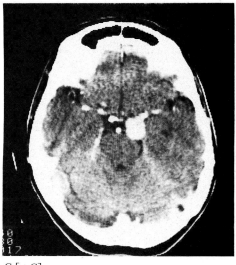

C [+C]

Case 58

Female, aged 89 years.
Several years' history of right third nerve palsy.

Q: This CT scan shows enhancing lesions on either
    side of the pituitary fossa. The most likely
    diagnosis is:

    i   Multiple meningiomas.
    ii Multiple neurofibromas.
    iii Aneurysms.
    iv Multiple granulomas.
    v   Metastases.

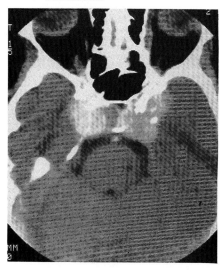

[+C]

Case 59

Male, aged 5 years.
Eleven-week history of visual difficulties.

Q: What diagnosis is suggested by this plain film and
    CT scan?

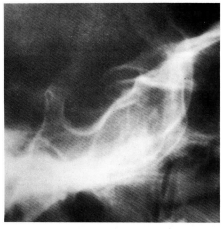

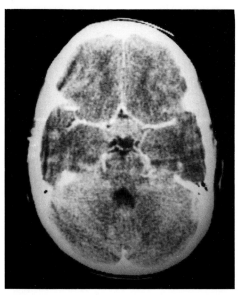

A

B [+C]

Case 58   Multiple meningiomas

All of these possible diagnoses have to be considered for multiple lesions in this location. The enhancement is rather too prominent to suggest neurofibromas, and aneurysms should show considerably more enhancement (*see* Case 57). Granulomas are certainly a possibility, but the history seems unduly long for this. Plain films or angiography could shed more light on this diagnosis, but careful assessment of the CT scan reveals thickening of the anterior clinoid processes and adjacent posterior walls of the orbits. Some calcification is present within the mass lying to the right of the sella. The bone thickening is the typical response at the base of meningiomas (enostosis) and calcification is also a feature of these lesions. (*See also* Cases 2 and 72.)

Carotid-cavernous fistulae are found in this region. Enhancement is more prominent than this and clinical examination would reveal a bruit over a protruding eye (proptosis).

Case 59   Optic chiasm glioma

The pituitary fossa shows a scalloping of its anterior superior margin. This is the region of the sulcus chiasmaticus and tuberculum sella. This sulcus may be prominent in children but never to this extent. There is also some undercutting of the anterior clinoids. These changes are not unlike those of the 'J-shaped' sella seen in aqueduct stenosis (*see* Case 5) and these appearances can be difficult to distinguish. The changes are very suggestive of a tumour of the optic chiasm producing pressure erosion of the adjacent bone. The CT scan confirms this. The suprasellar cistern is largely obliterated by a mildly enhancing lesion lying within the outline of the circle of Willis.

Optic chiasm glioma is a low-grade tumour found almost exclusively in children. Many cases are associated with neurofibromatosis (*see* Case 10). The lesion may extend into the orbits via the optic nerves producing enlargement of the optic foramen (*see Figure 36*). Angiography may show tumour circulation in the more aggressive lesions and MRI may be helpful in delineating the extent of infiltration. Visual loss is a prominent feature and slowly progressive. The principal differential diagnoses include benign neuromas in this area and hypothalamic glioma, but the finding of erosion of the sulcus chiasmaticus on plain films effectively excludes other diagnoses.

Case 60

Male, aged 74 years.
One-month history of headache and opthalmoplegia.

Q: On the basis of these plain-film changes, which of
these diagnoses would you consider most likely?

    i   Pituitary tumour.
    ii   Metastatic deposit.
    iii Chordoma.
    iv   Meningioma.

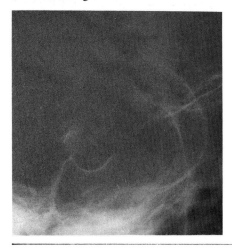

Case 61

Male aged 31 years.
Recurrent sinusitis for 5 years.

Q: This image is part of a series of plain films of the
paranasal sinuses. The pituitary fossa is enlarged
but there was no clinical evidence of pituitary
endocrine dysfunction, visual disturbance or
headaches. What other diagnosis should be
considered?

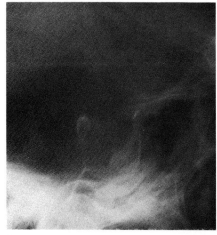

A

Case 60   Metastatic disease

This lateral skull film shows bone destruction without sclerosis involving the anterior part of the pituitary fossa, the tuberculum sella and posterior part of the anterior fossa floor. The remains of the pituitary fossa are not enlarged, so the appearances would not suggest an intrinsic pituitary lesion. Meningioma commonly shows evidence of bone involvement but when this is at the skull base then the response is primarily one of sclerosis (enostosis) rather than erosion. Chordoma in the skull invariably arises more posteriorly than this, from the clivus, and is usually associated with calcification (*see* Case 87). Benign lesions, such as neuroma or fibrous dysplasia, may affect the sphenoid bone, but these produce well-defined and marginated defects. This lesion is ill-defined and suggests a rapidly growing invasive process. Such an appearance may be produced by local extension of a primary carcinoma in the adjacent nasopharynx, or a metastatic deposit from a remote primary. In this case a mass was present in the nasopharynx on direct inspection. This was biopsied and showed highly malignant cells, probably metastatic.

Secondary deposits in the skull are common and present a wide variety of clinical manifestations. Metastases in the brain substance are discussed in Cases 3 and 43).

Case 61   Empty sella

It is becoming increasingly recognized that many normal individuals have varying degrees of extension of the subarachnoid space into the pituitary fossa. The pituitary gland then lies as a flattened structure in the lower fossa. The fossa is moderately enlarged—usually downwards, as in this case. These patients generally have no symptoms and the appearances are an incidental finding. The CSF extension can be demonstrated with air studies, CT or MRI. A CT scan on this patient is shown below. The low density of CSF can be seen within the fossa. This can be confused with a cystic pituitary tumour. Studies in the coronal plane with CT or MRI will usually demonstrate the continuity with suprasellar cisterns. In doubtful cases intrathecal air or contrast medium can be seen to enter the fossa.

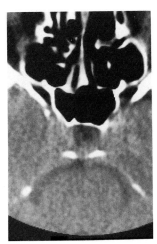

B

Coma

General considerations

Coma is a state of severely compromised consciousness. Several levels may be defined, depending on the degree of impairment. A diffuse reduction in neuronal activity is present in a comatose patient. This may be a reflection of a generalized brain disorder due to extrinsic or intrinsic causes, or some localized brain pathology whose nature is such as to be the cause of a widespread disruption of brain activity.

Extrinsic generalized causes of coma will not usually be evident on imaging techniques. These include such processes as diabetic coma, hepatic or renal failure, drug overdose, anoxia, etc. Occasionally some of these conditions may produce a non-specific cerebral oedema on CT.

Generalized intrinsic causes of coma may well have demonstrable manifestations on imaging techniques. These include such conditions as meningitis, encephalitis, subarachnoid haemorrhage and traumatic oedema. The postictal unconsciousness of epilepsy is usually of short duration and will only show an abnormality on imaging when some underlying structural cause is present.

Localized intrinsic causes of coma are particularly likely to be evident on imaging techniques. Practically any space-occupying intracranial lesion, including hydrocephalus, can result in coma. However, most of these would have symptoms and signs of developing intracranial pathology for some time and coma would only be seen at an advanced stage of the disease. Acute cerebral trauma, whether resulting in oedema, intracerebral or extracerebral haemorrhage, is an important and potentially treatable cause of coma. Spontaneous intracerebral haemorrhage or infarction are also readily demonstrated by imaging techniques and may be amenable to treatment.

A detailed history (from witnesses) and thorough physical examination will usually help indicate whether further investigation is required. A wide variety of biochemical or hormonal tests may be needed. The presence of tremor or flap will usually indicate a metabolic cause. Fever or neck stiffness will suggest meningitis or subarachnoid haemorrhage. The presence of papilloedema, unilateral limb signs or cranial nerve signs all suggest focal lesions and CT is mandatory. Signs of coning, i.e., fixed pupils with or without loss of ocular movements, and a deteriorating level of consciousness indicate serious raised intracranial pressure of a generalized or focal nature and urgent CT is indicated. A history of trauma is also a vital indication for CT in comatose patients. Plain skull films may reveal significant fractures or intracranial air.

The principal causes of coma with imaging manifestations are listed below. The first eight are described on the following pages.

Infarction
Cerebral oedema
Brainstem haemorrhage
Acute subdural haematoma
Extradural haematoma
Haemorrhagic tumour
Hydrocephalus
Traumatic intracerebral haemorrhage
Chronic subdural haematoma (Case 7)
Subarachnoid haemorrhage (Case 13)
Encephalitis (Case 15)
Meningitis (Case 20)
Cerebral abscess (Case 17)
Intraventricular tumours (Case 18)
Venous infarction (Case 21)

Case 62

Female, age unknown.
Found unconscious at home.

Q: The CT scan below was obtained as an emergency
investigation. What is your diagnosis, and
how does the scan help in management of this
case? (There was no change after contrast
enhancement.)

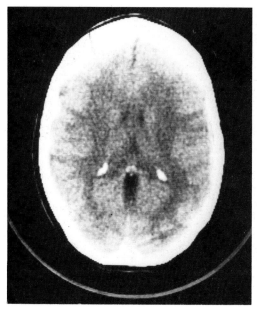

A

Case 62   Cerebral oedema

This is a common clinical situation: a comatose patient with little or no clinical history to aid the diagnosis. The patient may have a variety of systemic toxic conditions, but intracranial accidents such as haemorrhage or infarction need to be excluded. Infarction may require anticoagulation, and a haemorrhage may benefit from surgical evacuation.

In this case the scan shows small compressed ventricles and the white matter shows a general reduction in density which is partly patchy. These changes may be due to a space-occupying lesion higher up in the brain but other slices showed no evidence of this. The changes are due to generalized cerebral swelling or cerebral oedema. This is a non-specific response to a variety of factors. Generalized oedema such as this may be the result of overwhelming infection such as meningitis or encephalitis, cerebral trauma, venous occlusion (*see* Case 21) or systemic disorders such as drugs, renal failure, toxaemia of pregnancy, etc. In this case the cause was never established as the patient soon succumbed and a post-mortem was not performed. The cerebral oedema might have responded to plasma expanding fluids, steroids or craniotomy and decompression.

Two further examples of cerebral oedema are illustrated below. Image B shows generalized cerebral swelling following trauma with obliteration of the basal cisterns. Image C shows focal oedema in the left temporal lobe with mass effect. The plain-scan changes are typically confined to the white matter and are indistinguishable from other non-enhancing focal processes such as certain tumours and infections (*see* Cases 15 and 71). Angiography would show localized displacement of vessels in focal oedema or a general reduction in cerebral blood flow where the process is generalized.

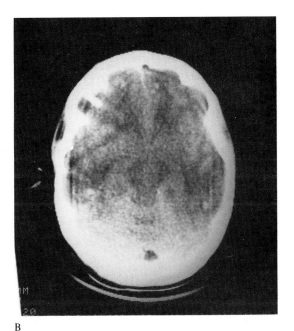

B

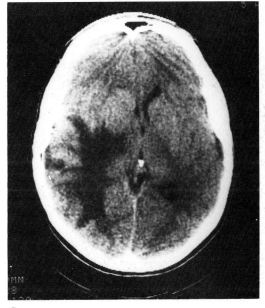

C

Case 63

Male, aged 5 days.
Respiratory depression and impaired vital signs.
Increasing head circumference.

Q: A plain skull film and cranial ultrasound examination were performed and are shown below (images A and B). What diagnosis can be made?

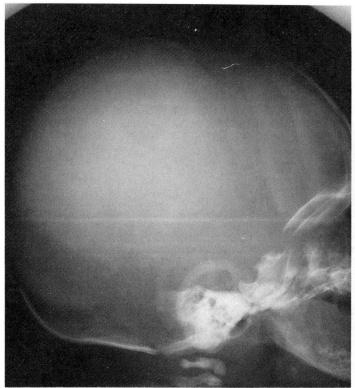

A

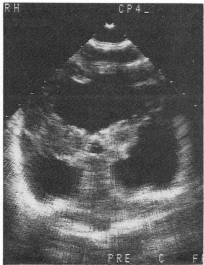

B

Case 63   Acute hydrocephalus

The plain skull film shows wide splaying of the cranial sutures consistent with raised intracranial pressure. The ultrasound examination has been obtained through the anterior fontanelle in the coronal plane (*see Figure 49*). This study shows wide dilatation of the lateral ventricles and their temporal horns. The third ventricle lying between them is also dilated. Scans in other planes suggested that the fourth ventricle was also dilated.

Hydrocephalus results from a wide range of causes and can present acutely with severe headache or progressive coma. Cases of hydrocephalus can be broadly divided into two groups. In non-communicating (internal) hydrocephalus, the dilated ventricular system does not have a proper communication with the subarachnoid cisterns. The ventricles are dilated but the basal cisterns are not. Intraventricular blood, tumours or congenital stenosis are the principal causes of this type of hydrocephalus. Communicating hydrocephalus (external) is characterized by free communication between the ventricles and subarachnoid spaces, and the obstruction lies within the basal cisterns or Sylvian fissures, at the tentorial hiatus, or over the convexity. The ventricles are dilated, as are the subarachnoid cisterns, the latter in a distribution dependent on the point of obstruction. This type of hydrocephalus may be caused by obliteration of the cisterns following meningitis, subarachnoid haemorrhage, trauma or carcinomatous invasion. Examples of these various types of hydrocephalus are described in Cases 5, 20 and 90.

The present case shows dilatation of all four ventricles. The obstruction is therefore likely to be at the outlet of the fourth ventricle or basal cisterns. A CT scan would probably be helpful in demonstrating whether or not the basal cisterns were dilated, although this may have little bearing on management in this case. As a general rule, where neonatal ultrasound satisfactorily demonstrates the size of all four ventricles in a case of hydrocephalus, then CT is not usually necessary.

An important form of hydrocephalus may be encountered in young children. This is a type of communicating hydrocephalus where the head circumference is increased and the ventricles are dilated, with excess fluid in the basal cisterns and over the hemispheres. The CT appearances are rather like those of atrophy (*see* Case 89), but are probably due to defective resorption of CSF at the sagittal sinus. The condition is usually benign and self-limiting. A case is shown below in images C and D.

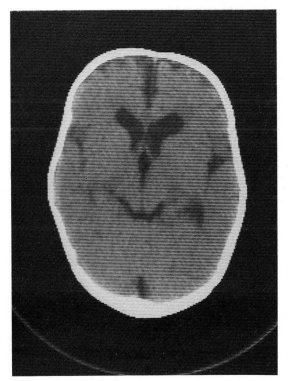

C

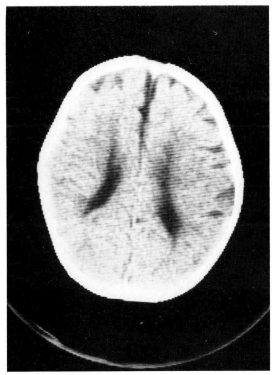

D

Case 64

Male, aged 18.
Semi-conscious since accident on motorcycle.

Q: This plain film was obtained. What is the special
     significance of the vault fracture?

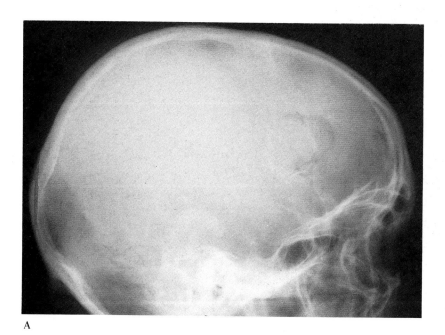

A

Case 64   Depressed fracture/traumatic intracerebral haemorrhage

This lateral skull film shows an irregular fractured area in the frontal region. In some parts the fracture shows dense lines. This is due to bone fragments being rotated or overlapped and almost invariably indicates that some of the bone fragments are depressed inwards. This is a potentially serious complication of skull fractures, as the bone fragments may damage blood vessels, dura or the brain itself. Cases that show this feature should have a CT scan to assess the extent of any associated intracraniai damage. The CT scan on this patient is shown below (B). There is some oedema and focal haemorrhage in the right frontal lobe. The depressed bone fragment can be seen just lateral to this.

Traumatic focal haemorrhage is common and is often found in patients without depressed fractures.

The commonest sites for this change are in the tips of the frontal or temporal lobes where the brain is enclosed by a bony pocket. When a head injury is sustained the brain is often pressed against bone on the side opposite to that of the point of impact. Such a case is illustrated in C. This patient sustained a blow on the back of the head and this has produced a focal haemorrhage with some oedema in the tip of the right temporal lobe. This mechanism of damage is known as 'contrecoup'.

Traumatic intracerebral haemorrhage may not be evident immediately after the injury and several days can elapse before the blood becomes obvious on CT. Haemorrhage within the cerebral substance is frequently associated with extracerebral haematomas of extradural or subdural type.

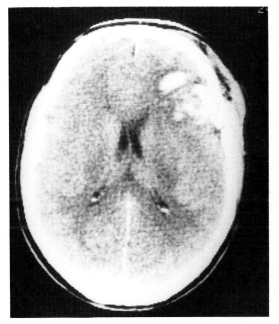

B

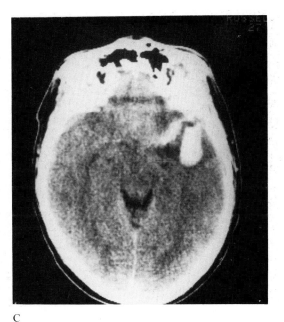

C

Case 65

Female, aged 25 years.
Semi-comatose following head injury.

Q: The CT scanner was being serviced and an arteriogram was obtained. What does this show, and how might this appear on CT?

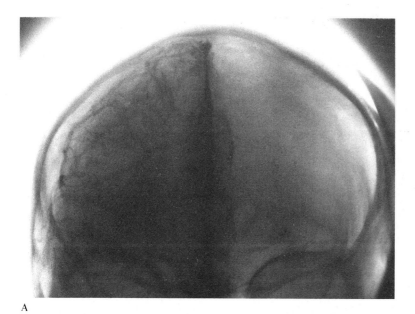

A

Case 65   Acute subdural haematoma

Before CT scanning became widely available radiology departments spent a substantial amount of time performing angiography on head-injured patients. The purpose of this (as with CT) was to look for potentially treatable lesions such as haematomas. This case provides an example of such a situation. The midline vessels are displaced to the patient's left side, indicating a mass effect on the right. The cause for this mass effect is evident on closer inspection. The cortical vessels over the convexity are displaced away from the vault over quite a wide area but remain parallel to it. This appearance is characteristic of a fluid collection in the subdural space. This could be a haematoma from trauma or (rarely) from an aneurysm. Alternatively, a subdural collection of pus (*see* Case 19) could produce this appearance. Acute subdural collections are characteristically fairly shallow and widely spread over the hemisphere, in distinction from extradural collections which are more localized (*see* Case 66). Image B is from a CT study in a patient with an acute subdural haematoma and shows the characteristic high-density layer of blood over the hemisphere and some midline shift. The layer of blood may be thinly spread and difficult to see. The mass effect is usually evident however. In this case there is also some generalized swelling of the right hemisphere and compression of the right lateral ventricle. The left lateral ventricle is dilated and contains blood in its occipital horn.

The changes on the arteriogram and CT scan are common consequences of head trauma. These patients may show a variety of symptoms and signs, including headache, coma, weakness, seizures, etc. Many of them deteriorate rapidly and investigation will have to be undertaken as an emergency. Occasionally, however, the presence of a haematoma goes unnoticed in the acute phase and the lesion may go on to become a low-density chronic subdural collection. (*See* Cases 7 and 32.)

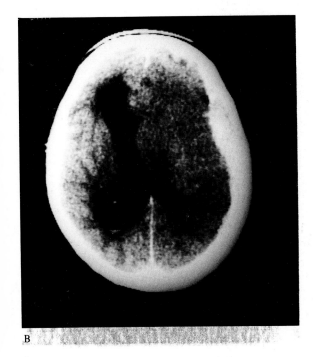

B

Case 66

Female, aged 23 years.
Head injury while pillion rider on motorcycle.
Brief loss of consciousness and recovery, now
conscious level deteriorating again.

Q: This plain film was obtained. What pathology
      does it show? Does this patient warrant further
      investigation?

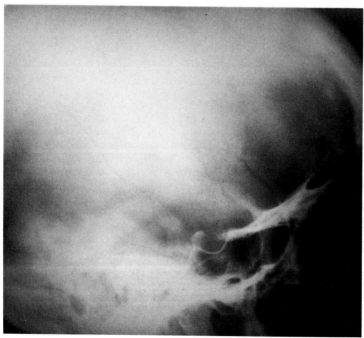

A

Case 66   Acute extradural haematoma

Many patients with head injury are rendered unconscious for a short period and rapidly recover. No further investigation is required if they continue to improve and neurological signs do not develop. The presence of amnesia of more than 10 minutes' duration, or a significant scalp laceration are indications for plain skull radiography. Patients with fluctuating levels of consciousness, severe headache, neurological signs, evidence of depressed fracture, or fracture of the skull base will probably require a CT scan to assess the extent of possible intracranial damage.

In this case the plain film shows a fracture crossing the left temporoparietal area. This in itself is not a serious problem. However, the story of initial brief loss of consciousness followed by recovery, then further deterioration, is very suggestive of a developing intracranial haematoma, possibly of extradural type. This extracerebral bleed occurs between the vault and the dura and is usually the result of a laceration of the middle meningeal artery. Fractures in this site cross the path of this vessel and may cause it to be torn. The accumulation of blood is more rapid than with subdural haematoma (see Case 65), but because of the tight adherence of the dura to the vault the collection cannot spread widely. This produces a lentiform collection of high-density material on CT scan. This patient's scan is shown below (image B) and the lentiform high-density collection is shown in the left temporal area. There is marked midline shift. This is the commonest site for these collections but occasionally examples may be encountered in other sites where meningeal vessels occur, for example, in the posterior fossa, frontal region, etc. The majority of these lesions present acutely, but very occasionally an example may be seen where the injury occurred days or weeks before, and the collection now shows areas of mixed density as blood products start to disintegrate and resorb.

Some patients may demonstrate a degree of hemiparesis due to focal compression of the underlying hemispheres. Angiography would be expected to show a lentiform displacement of vessels away from the vault, very similar to the arteriographic changes in chronic subdural haematoma (see Case 32).

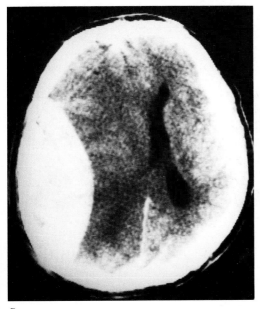

B

Case 67

Female, aged 44 years.
Deeply unconscious since craniotomy for aneurysm
clipping.

Q: This CT scan was obtained. What diagnosis
   would you consider?

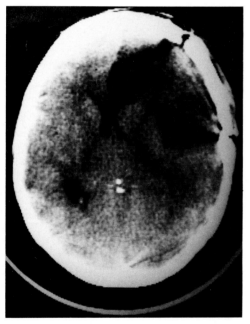

A

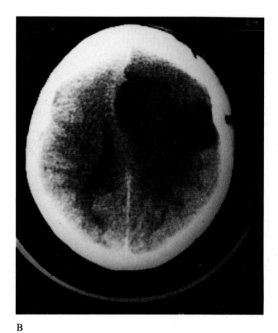

B

Case 67   Cerebral infarction (postoperative)

Scans A and B show a fairly well-defined low-density area in the right frontal region with displacement of ventricular structures to the left. The craniotomy flap can be seen overlying this area. Areas of swelling or oedema are quite common following surgery but this appearance is excessive. Clipping of aneurysms can be associated with complications. Spasm, when severe, can lead to areas of ischaemia or infarction, but in this case misplacement of the aneurysm clip had resulted in occlusion of the anterior cerebral artery and ischaemia in the middle cerebral artery territory. The appearances on the CT scans are due to infarction in these territories. This degree of swelling is unusual in

infarction, but the particular circumstances of the ischaemia may have produced concomitant venous 'hold-up' leading to oedema.

Infarction may also be the result of trauma: whiplash or direct injuries of the neck may cause internal damage to the carotid or vertebral arteries leading to occlusion or distal embolism.

This patient recovered and finally left hospital with a moderate neurological deficit. A further scan 5 months later shows that the swelling has been replaced by well-defined atrophic areas and focal dilatation of the frontal horn—common long term sequelae of major infarcts.

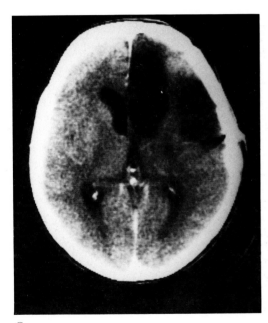

C

Case 68

Male, aged 64.
Known hypertensive, found unconscious at the bottom of garden.

Q: There were no signs of head injury and a skull radiograph showed no fracture. What does this CT scan show?

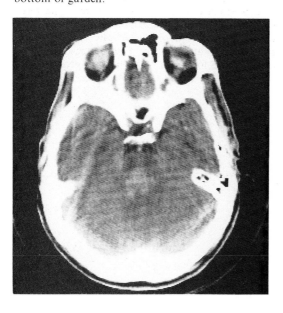

Case 69

Male, aged 48.
Sudden onset of severe headache and rapid loss of consciousness.
Personality change for 3 months previously.

Q: The CT scan shows a haemorrhage in the left frontal lobe. Do you feel that the diagnosis is now complete?

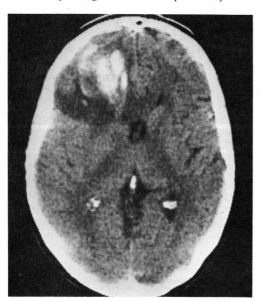

A

Case 68   Pontine haemorrhage

Clearly the circumstances of the discovery raised the question of a head injury, and although there were no external signs a CT scan was still indicated to ascertain the cause of coma. The scan shows a raised density area within the brainstem, the slice having been taken at the level of the pons. The image is mildly degraded as the patient's conscious level lightened during the scan and some movement was present. The density is irregular in outline and is insufficiently dense to be calcification. Its appearance is therefore consistent with a haemorrhage. This is a fairly common site for intracranial haemorrhage and, because of the presence of vital structures, the outcome is often fatal. Hydrocephalus is commonly associated. The bleed may be the result of a local lesion such as aneurysm, tumour or AVM. Trauma can also produce haemorrhage at this site. This patient had been hypertensive for years and this was probably the underlying cause.

Case 69   Haemorrhage into tumour

The high-density area in the left frontal lobe is consistent with a fresh intracerebral haemorrhage with some surrounding oedema. There is some compression and backward displacement of the frontal horns. The position of this bleed is not really appropriate for intracerebral extension of a bleed from an aneurysm on the anterior cerebral circulation, being a little too far laterally placed. The patient was not known to be hypertensive and this would be an unusual site for this source anyway. There was no change after contrast enhancement. The patient recovered rapidly and surgical decompression was considered unnecessary. The story of previous personality change began to emerge and further follow-up was considered essential. Four weeks later an enhanced scan (image B) shows the haemorrhage to have cleared and the site is now occupied by a large low-density lesion with an irregular enhancing margin consistent with a glioma (*see* Case 1). Haemorrhage into an underlying tumour is not uncommon and should always be kept in mind in such cases. Some benign haematomas may, however, develop an enhancing margin as they resolve, but in these the mass effect gets less rather than more and the oedema would have subsided (*see* Case 76).

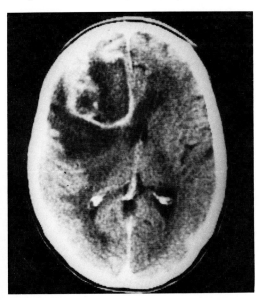

B [+C]

Sensory disorders

General considerations

This chapter covers sensory disorders originating in the cranial cavity which produce disturbance of sensation in the limbs and trunk. Abnormal vision and disorders of smell are also included here, but sensory disorders related to cranial nerves below the tentorium are covered in the chapter on the cerebellum and related structures. The various sensory modalities have complex pathways and disorder patterns; the reader is referred to detailed neurology texts for a full description. This is particularly relevant for the clinical distinction of peripheral or cord-based sensory loss from causes arising within the brain.

The principal sensory pathways from the trunk and limbs pass up through the brainstem, reaching the thalamus and internal capsule via the cerebral peduncles. From here the fibres radiate out to the sensory cortex (postcentral, parietal). The more deeply placed lesions in this system will produce extensive sensory loss on the contralateral side of the body. Lesions in the cortex may simply affect an arm or leg only. The sensory and motor pathways are closely associated, therefore both are often involved. Lesions in the thalamus usually produce a marked sensory loss, often with some hemiparesis, and occasionally a burning pain, all on the opposite side of the body. Brainstem lesions tend to affect pain and temperature

sensation, often with half the face involved and the opposite side of the body. The need for intracranial imaging techniques in patients with sensory disorders of the trunk and limbs is dependent on the clinical assessment of the likely level of involvement. Mononeuropathies are usually characterized by involvement of all sensory modalities in the distribution of the affected peripheral nerve. Involvement at root level produces a sensory change in a dermatomal distribution. Cord involvement may produce a variety of combinations of motor and sensory loss, the latter being of mixed pain and temperature, position or vibration sense type. A sensory level is often present on the trunk. Other sensory patterns of agnosia, unilateral inattention, hemianaesthesia or dysaesthesia suggest an intracranial lesion; a full assessment including plain skull films and CT or MRI will usually be required. If a vascular lesion is suspected angiography may be needed.

Visual loss may be due to a lesion at any level from the cornea to the occipital cortex. Lesions affecting one eye only may be within the eye itself, or its optic nerve or artery. Transient loss of vision in one eye due to ischaemia is common in older patients with embolic episodes (amaurosis fugax, *see* Case 48). Optic neuritis may occur on its own or as part of multiple sclerosis, and the diagnosis is usually evident on history taking and fundoscopy; it may also be bilateral. Optic

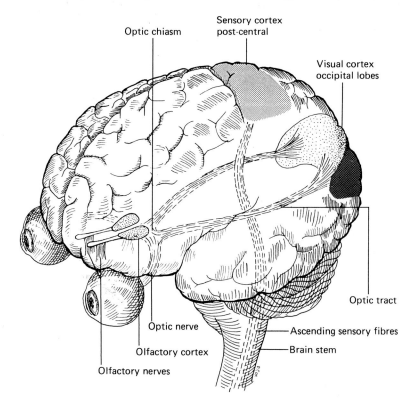

Optic chiasm

Sensory cortex post-central

Visual cortex occipital lobes

Optic nerve

Olfactory cortex

Olfactory nerves

Optic tract

Ascending sensory fibres

Brain stem

atrophy has a variety of causes, including toxic or familial conditions with no significant imaging manifestations. Multiple sclerosis may produce optic atrophy and, as in the case of optic neuritis, may be associated with demonstrable lesions elsewhere. These may be revealed by CT or MRI scanning (*see* Case 70). Pressure on the optic nerves by masses inside the orbit, optic foramen, or along the basal cisterns and chiasm can also lead to optic atrophy, and such lesions can be readily demonstrated with imaging techniques. Visual field disorders affecting both eyes may occur as a result of damage to both eyes or both optic nerves, but in this chapter only lesions affecting the optic chiasm, optic radiations or visual occipital cortex are covered. Lesions involving the chiasm, including intrinsic lesions such as glioma, or extrinsic such as pituitary masses, broadly cause bilateral loss of the temporal fields of vision. Homonymous hemianopia is caused by lesions in the optic radiation or occipital lobe. Other complex forms of field loss are encountered. Depending on whether clinical assessment suggests the lesion to be in front or behind the chiasm, then imaging techniques should be chosen to suit the likely location of the lesion. A lateral skull film (to exclude a pituitary mass) should be obtained in all cases of visual failure who do not have obvious ocular lesions. Anterior lesions will require high quality CT or detailed plain films of the optic foraminae and sellar area, possibly with tomography. High-resolution CT, perhaps with intrathecal contrast enhancement, may be needed to define small lesions. Posteriorly placed lesions, however, may be defined with CT or MRI.

Disorders of smell are uncommon. Hallucinations of inappropriate smells may be a manifestation of temporal lobe epilepsy, schizophrenia or depression. Loss of the sense of smell may be due to infections or allergies in the nasal sinus or dental areas. However, traumatic lesions of the cribriform plate, anterior fossa meningiomas or, rarely, olfactory neuroblastoma can also cause loss of the sense of smell.

The diagram opposite shows the sensory pathways discussed in this section.

In the absence of obvious causes in the nasal passages, sinuses or teeth, olfactory disturbances may require detailed plain films and tomography of the anterior fossa floor and CT scanning.

The list below is incomplete but provides some idea of the many causes of sensory loss. The first seven cases are described on the following pages.

Sensory cortex infarction
Occipital haemorrhage
Occipital infarction
Olfactory meningioma
Multiple sclerosis
Intrinsic tumour
Optic chiasm compression
Brainstem tumours (Case 78)
Posterior fossa masses (Case 79)
Basilar artery occlusion
Larger aneurysms (Case 83)
Metastases (Case 41)

Case 70

Female, aged 44 years.
Six-year history of attacks of various neurological
disorders including visual loss. Currently presenting
with sensory loss at several sites in the limbs.

Q: These T2-weighted MRI scans were obtained.
    What is your diagnosis?

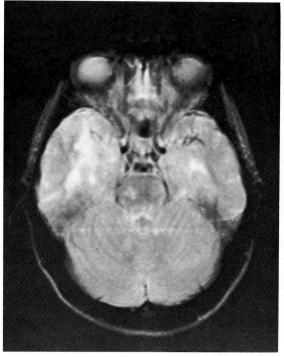

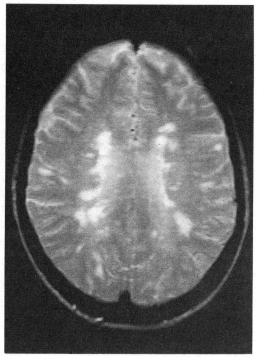

A   B

Case 70   Multiple sclerosis

Image A is an axial slice through the cerebellum and orbits. A number of high-signal (long T2) areas are shown in the cerebellum and brainstem. Further lesions are present in the temporal lobes. Image B is a slice taken through the cerebral hemispheres just above the lateral ventricles. A large number of high-signal areas are shown in the white matter. The appearances are consistent with demyelination due to multiple sclerosis.

Multiple sclerosis is a common disease of unknown aetiology in which plaques of demyelination occur throughout the nervous system. These occur acutely producing a variety of neurological deficits. Both brain and spinal cord may be involved and optic nerve manifestations are particularly common. Visual loss, ataxia, weakness, etc. may all be encountered at different phases in the illness. The lesions often clear with relief of symptoms, but over a period of years the neurological deficits accumulate. Prior to the advent of MRI and CT scanning, imaging techniques had

little to offer in the diagnosis of multiple sclerosis.

The changes on MRI shown in this case are typical of demyelination. T1-weighted sequences show low-signal areas. The lesions are typically periventricular in distribution and mostly in the white matter. Lesions may also be demonstrated in the spinal cord. Similar appearances can be produced by other forms of demyelination, multiple infarcts, etc and small foci of high signal must be considered normal in patients over 60. Acute MS plaques may show enhancement with gadolinium. The diagnosis of MS is essentially a clinical one which can be supported by MRI. The lesions shown on MRI correlate well with the clinical manifestations and MRI may be helpful in monitoring the disease and indicating prognosis. CT scanning may also show these plaques, but is considerably less sensitive than MRI. Low-density areas are shown in such a case below (C). Some cases show quite marked contrast enhancement.

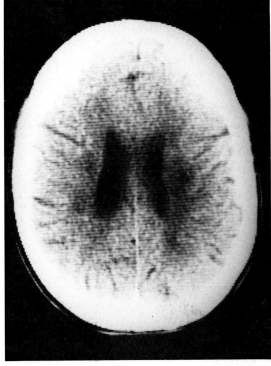

C

Case 71

Male, aged 34 years.
Two-month history of left hemiparaesthesia and left hemiparesis.
Gradual onset.

Q: What features are present in this case which suggest that the lesion shown on the CT scans is *not* due to infarction?

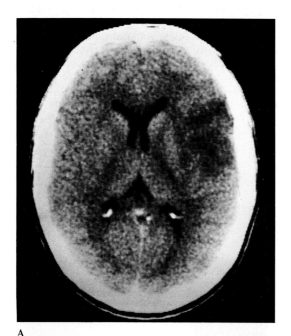

A

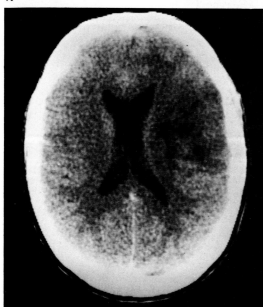

B

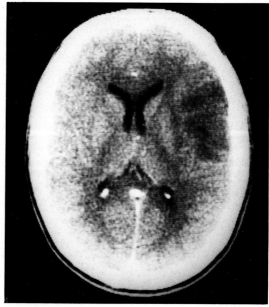

C [+C]

Case 71   Low-grade astrocytoma

Images A and B are unenhanced and show a roughly wedge-shaped area within the territory of the right middle cerebral artery. The slice at the higher level (B) shows that the lesion extends into the corona radiata; this explains the sensory component in the patient's symptoms (the sensory afferent pathways pass up to the cortex via the corona radiata). Scan C shows no change after contrast enhancement. The appearances bear a strong resemblance to a partial infarction in the middle cerebral artery territory. However, two important features are against this diagnosis: first, the duration of symptoms and gradual onset are very unlike infarction (see Case 22); secondly, the scans show mild midline shift away from the lesion and slight posterior displacement of the right trigone. These latter characteristics point to a mass effect, a feature seen infrequently in infarction, and then only in the early stages. The appearances are due to a low-grade astrocytoma.

This lesion can present considerable problems in diagnosis. Related forms include the calcified or cystic astrocytoma (see Cases 39 and 46). This type can mimic encephalitis, venous infarction, granulomata, etc., and unless a biopsy is performed, only serial scanning over several years will confirm the slowly progressive neoplastic nature of the lesion. MRI can show such lesions but it is as yet unclear whether it can provide an earlier definitive diagnosis than serial CT. Angiography is often performed and is usually inconclusive. The absence of significant enhancement on CT makes the finding of appreciable tumour vessels unlikely, and angiography invariably shows only displaced arteries and veins around the lesion. This patient had an arteriogram which is shown below (D). The branches of the middle cerebral artery above the Sylvian fissure are displaced downwards (arrows) and stretched by the local mass effect of the tumour. There is no tumour circulation.

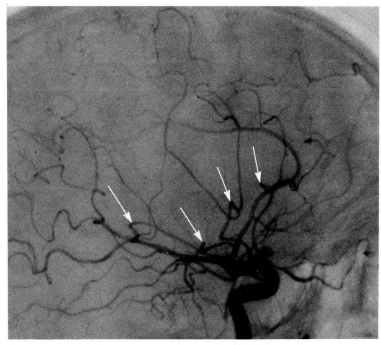

D

Case 72

Female, aged 40 years.
Fifteen-month history of progressive loss of sense of smell.

Q: This plain film was part of a skull series obtained
    on this patient. What three important signs are
    present?

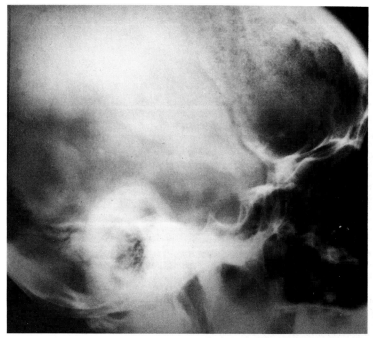

A

Case 72   Olfactory groove meningioma

This lateral skull film shows erosion of the dorsum sella consistent with longstanding raised intracranial pressure, or direct pressure from a lesion in the suprasellar area. Further forward some areas of calcification are seen over the lower part of the anterior fossa. These two signs suggest that a calcified mass is present at this site. Furthermore, just below this, the floor of the anterior fossa shows bony thickening. The latter feature is highly suggestive of a bony enostosis at the point of attachment of meningioma.

Image B shows the CT scan on this patient. The well-defined, calcified and enhancing tumour is shown just above the anterior fossa floor in the midline. This is one of the classic sites for meningioma and calcification is commonly seen within these tumours. For further descriptions of meningiomas *see* Cases 2 and 28. Any mass at this site is likely to cause a disturbance of the sense of smell by involvement of the olfactory cortex or nerves, but meningioma is the most likely cause.

The CT appearance of meningioma is usually fairly typical, with a well-defined raised density area on the plain scans at a characteristic site. Enhancement shows a marked uniform further increase in density. Some tumours are atypical and show areas of necrosis producing a very irregular pattern, but the meningeal location should continue to suggest the true diagnosis. Occasionally meningiomas are very heavily calcified and can be mistaken for bone tumours arising from the vault. Rarely a flat plate-like area of tumour is encountered. This is called 'meningioma-en-plaque' and can be very difficult to see where it lies along the floor of the middle cranial fossa. Primary intracranial lymphoma can produce a very similar appearance to meningioma but is invariably located within the cerebral substance (*see* Case 93). Granulomas are rather rare but can produce a similar pattern of enhancement, especially in the basal cisterns (*see* Case 12). Metastases can occasionally show raised density on plain scan and uniform enhancement similar to meningioma but are usually within the cerebral substance. Metastases from bowel tumours or malignant melanoma are most likely to produce this CT appearance (*see* Case 43).

Image C shows a carotid arteriogram from a patient with a meningioma arising from the tentorium and producing compression of the brainstem. It is being supplied by the tentorial branch of the meningohypophyseal artery—a small vessel arising from the carotid siphon (arrow). This vessel supplies an ill-defined blush behind the carotid siphon.

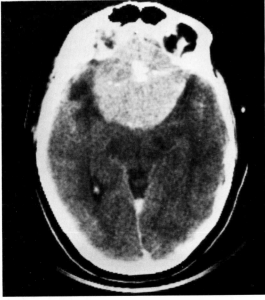

B [+C]

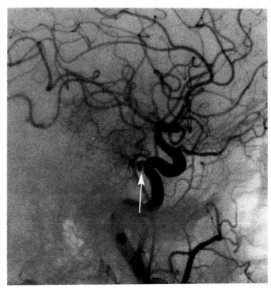

C

Case 73

Male, aged 43 years.
One-year history of deteriorating vision.
Bitemporal hemianopia.

Q: This sagittal T1-weighted spin-echo sequence
MRI scan was obtained. What is your diagnosis?

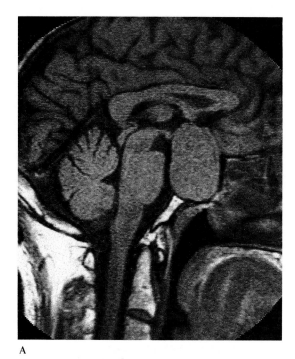

A

Case 73   Suprasellar extension of pituitary tumour

A large lesion is seen rising upwards from the pituitary fossa which is clearly considerably enlarged. The lesion is of intermediate signal and extends up through the anterior third ventricle to the level of the foramen of Munro. Such upward extension can produce pressure on adjacent structures such as the optic chiasm (hence the visual signs), arteries, other cranial nerves or the ventricular system (with consequent hydrocephalus).

Larger pituitary lesions commonly extend beyond the confines of the pituitary fossa. Consequent deterioration of vision may require urgent neurosurgical intervention, and there may be no appreciable endocrine manifestations. Pituitary lesions may also extend laterally, causing compression of the IIIrd, IVth or VIth cranial nerves within the cavernous sinuses with defective ocular movements. Such extension beyond the fossa can be well visualized on MRI as shown here. Coronal plane images will demonstrate lateral extension. High-resolution CT with intravenous enhancement will also demonstrate this complication (*see* image B). Angiography will show lateral extension by lateral displacement of the carotid siphons, or upward extension by elevation of the horizontal portion of the anterior cerebral artery (arrow, image C).

Other possible diagnoses for the appearance in image A include craniopharyngioma, aneurysms, etc. (*see* Cases 56 and 57).

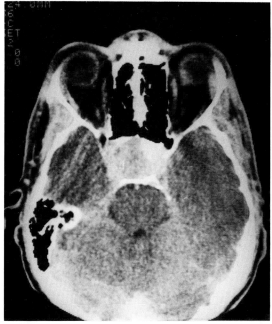

B [+C]

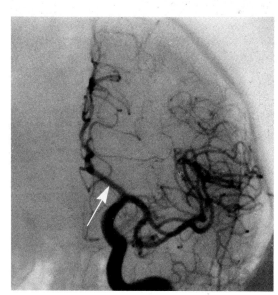

C

Case 74

Female, aged 48 years.
Sudden onset of right-sided visual disturbance.
Right hemianopia.

Q: This CT scan was obtained. There was no change
    after contrast enhancement. The most likely
    diagnosis is:

    i   Encephalitis.
    ii   Low-grade astrocytoma.
    iii Infarction in territory of posterior cerebral
        artery.
    iv Cerebral haemorrhage.
    v   Venous infarction.

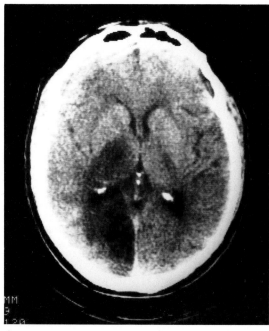

A

Case 74   Infarction: posterior cerebral artery territory

The scan demonstrates an extensive low-density area in the posterior part of the left hemisphere. The trigone and choroid are not compressed or displaced so there is no evident mass effect. The lesion also affects most of the left thalamus. Fresh haemorrhage presents high density on CT and is therefore not a possibility here Venous infarctions are often haemorrhagic and tend to occur in the upper hemisphere. This posterior location would be a most unusual site for encephalitis (*see* Case 15). Low-grade astrocytomas could present this appearance but usually show some mass effect (*see* Case 71). The history and distribution of the lesion is characteristic of extensive infarction in the territory of the left posterior cerebral artery. The diagram with Case 24 shows the broad territories supplied by the major supratentorial arteries. The posterior cerebral artery supplies the occipital lobe with its visual cortex, the posterior and inferior aspect of the temporal lobe and provides some deep branches to the thalamus. The latter structure is usually spared in infarcts of this territory. The extent of the lesion depends on the number of branches involved and only small areas may be involved. In the patient illustrated below (B) only the left temporal lobe branches are involved and the occipital cortex is spared (vision was unaffected). For a general discussion on infarction *see* Case 22.

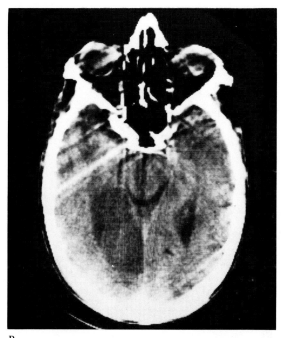

B

Case 75

Female, aged 73 years.
Six-day history of right hemianaesthesia.

Q: What features are present on this CT scan? There
      was no change after contrast enhancement.

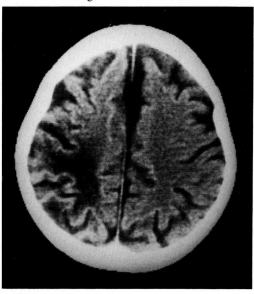

Case 76

Female, aged 29 years.
Eleven-day history of visual disturbance.
Found to have right homonymous hemianopia.

Q: The pre- and post-contrast CT scans are shown
      below. What is your differential diagnosis?

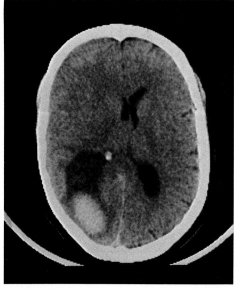

A   B [+C]

Case 75   Cortical infarction

The scan shows generalized widening of sulci and the interhemispheral fissure in keeping with the patient's age (*see* Case 89). In addition, there is a low density area in the white matter of the upper left cerebral hemisphere. The adjacent gyri are not displaced, so there is little or no mass effect. This represents an area of focal cerebral oedema or softening. Tumour is unlikely in the absence of mass effect and enhancement, but an early infiltrating glioma would have to be considered. The short history is very unlike a tumour except in the presence of a bleed (*see* Case 69). There was no history of trauma, surgery or radiation therapy. This would be a most unusual site for encephalitis.

The lesion is the result of cortical infarction. A small branch of the middle cerebral artery has been occluded distally and this area of focal ischaemia has ensued. Its position high in the hemisphere is close to the sensory and motor cortex around the central sulcus. This accounts for the sensory presentation (sensory stroke). If the lesion were more anteriorly placed, a motor disorder would probably have been the result. Small infarcts in the internal capsule or brainstem could also produce a major sensory deficit. Infarcts in the occipital cortex may produce a visual sensory disturbance (*see* Case 74).

Angiography may be normal in patients with more peripheral infarcts, particularly if performed some time after the event.

Case 76   Posthaemorrhagic cyst

Image A shows a well-defined low-density area in the left occipital pole causing forward displacement of the calcified choroid plexus and some midline shift to the right. Posteriorly the lesion contains an ill-defined area of raised density. Following contrast enhancement the whole lesion is delineated by a fine enhancing edge with little obvious surrounding oedema. Lesions in, or compressing the occipital lobe characteristically produce a hemianopia.

Several diagnostic possibilities have to be considered here. The lesion has an overall density slightly higher than CSF so it is probably cystic. The raised density area looks more like haemorrhage than calcification. It is possible therefore that this represents haemorrhage into a cystic tumour. An infarct that is this well defined would be old and therefore should have no mass effect. A variety of granulomatous lesions and metastatic disease would have to be considered.

The lesion was explored and found to be a resolving haematoma. A subsequent arteriogram showed a small AVM at the apex of the occipital lobe as the source of the bleed. This is a common trap for the unwary. As intracerebral haematomas resorb they often leave behind a cystic cavity, the wall of which may enhance for some months. The resulting CT appearance may readily be mistaken for all kinds of active pathology if the possibility of a preceding haemorrhage is not considered. Serial CT scanning may be helpful in cases where doubt exists. Perhaps the most helpful feature to distinguish this lesion from a glioma or abscess is that in this cyst there is usually little or no low density beyond the enhancing ring. Gliomas or abscesses usually show extensive oedema beyond the area of enhancement.

The posterior fossa and cranial nerves

General considerations

This section includes lesions arising in, or affecting, the cranial nerves, brainstem or cerebellum. Disorders of the first and second cranial nerves affecting smell or vision are covered in the chapter on sensory disorders; these are usually isolated from other cranial nerve signs and their causes are normally exclusively supratentorial. The symptoms and signs in this section fall into three broad categories which frequently occur in combination and are not mutually exclusive.

1. Cerebellar signs.
2. Brainstem signs.
3. Cranial nerve signs.

The cerebellum controls postural reflexes and muscular tone thereby maintaining general equilibrium. Voluntary movements are modified using a complex system of control enabling them to be performed smoothly, precisely and in a coordinated fashion. Failure of these cerebellar functions results in uncoordinated hand movements and gait ('ataxia'). Reduction in muscle tone, nystagmus, intention tremor and 'scanning' speech may also be encountered. These manifestations of cerebellar dysfunction may be the result of either intrinsic lesions such as infarction, tumour, etc., or other posterior fossa pathology causing compression or distortion of the cerebellum.

The brainstem contains: the nuclei for all the cranial nerves III to XII; the sensory and motor pathways running between the cerebral hemispheres, cerebellum and spinal cord; and also the reticular formation. The stem is compact, and even quite small lesions can have very dramatic and specific effects. A combination of a specific cranial nerve deficit and long tract signs can provide very accurate localization of an intrinsic or extrinsic brainstem lesion. The absence of long tract signs suggests the lesion may lie in the cranial nerve beyond the brainstem. The long motor tracts cross over in the medulla so that the contralateral element of cortical symptoms and signs is present for lesions above this level, and absent for those affecting the lower medulla. Disorders of the reticular formation affect consciousness and sleep.

The IIIrd, IVth and VIth cranial nerves are primarily concerned with ocular movements. A lesion of the IIIrd nerve will usually cause drooping of the eyelid (ptosis), dilated pupil, and varying degrees of failure of upward and/or medial movement of the eye. Pathology involving the VIth nerve prevents lateral eye movements. Disorders of the VIth nerve functions are the most common, followed by those of the IIIrd nerve. Pure lesions of the IVth nerve are very uncommon. The Vth cranial nerve is principally involved in facial sensation and the VIIth nerve with facial movements and some taste sensation anteriorly on the tongue. The VIIIth nerve has both cochlear (hearing) and vestibular (balance) components. The IXth and Xth nerves control coughing, phonation and swallowing. These nerves are also involved in pharyngeal reflexes and in taste sensation. The XIth nerve is partly involved in the functions of the IXth and Xth but also controls important functions in the shoulder muscles. The XIIth nerve has only one function, that is to control tongue movements.

These cranial nerves may be affected by pathology at any point along their course, from their point of origin in a brainstem nucleus, to the principal course of the nerve or at their point of effect. Consequently a wide variety of lesions can cause cranial nerve deficits. Intrinsic brainstem lesions such as multiple sclerosis, tumours, infarcts, haemorrhage or encephalitis will usually have long tract signs or other cranial nerves involved, thereby indicating the central nature of the pathology. Distortion of the stem by cerebellar and extra-axial masses or brain herniations may produce the same effect. The nerves may be affected along their course by neuromas, meningiomas, aneurysms or lesions such as metastases within the skull base. Raised intracranial pressure commonly results in medial and downward displacement of the medial temporal lobe through the tentorial hiatus with consequent compression of the IIIrd nerve.

The region under discussion here is affected by a number of conditions which do not have imaging manifestations. These include Bell's palsy, Ménière's syndrome and various toxic or drug-induced states together with diabetic neuropathies. Bell's palsy is a unilateral facial palsy of sudden onset. This latter feature with gradual recovery is typical; further investigation is rarely necessary. Trigeminal neuralgia is characterized by brief attacks of severe pain in the face. It generally occurs in older patients and is rarely associated with abnormal neurological signs. Some workers believe that all new cases should receive a CT scan since tumours such as meningioma or Schwannoma are found in some patients. Ménière's syndrome can be caused by a variety of lesions and shows recurrent vertigo attacks, often with hearing loss and tinnitus. The paroxysmal nature is typical in distinction from acoustic neuroma where the course is progressive. Acoustic neuroma must be considered in all older patients with progressive unilateral deafness that is not clearly otogenic; CT scanning is the technique of choice. Certain drugs, toxic states including virus infections, and systemic conditions such as diabetes may be associated with symptoms and signs referrable to the posterior fossa or cranial nerves.

A detailed history and neurological examination is essential in these patients as it is often possible to predict the likely site of the abnormality from this information. These areas are often difficult to assess by imaging techniques and a sound clinical assessment may go a long way towards limiting the possible sites and the extent of the investigations. Good plain films (including perhaps tomography) of the parasellar region and skull base are invaluable, and the ensuing cases will illustrate this point. Where MRI is available this is now generally accepted to be the most sensitive of the principal techniques for assessing likely lesions of the brainstem and cerebellum. CT is a close second best, but can be disappointing because of artefacts close to the skull base and in the posterior fossa. Intravenous contrast enhancement and high-resolution/narrow slices can significantly increase its performance in these cases. Intrathecally enhanced CT can provide exquisite delineation of certain lesions. Angiography can be helpful in lesions close to the sella or cavernous sinus, and in other situations outlined on the ensuing pages.

Some of the commoner lesions in the posterior fossa and cranial nerves with imaging manifestations are listed below. See also the section on sensory disorders.

Acoustic neuroma
Brainstem infarction
Brainstem glioma
Aneurysms
Basilar invagination
Chordoma of the clivus
Ependymoma
Trigeminal neuroma
Haemangioblastoma
Medulloblastoma
Cerebellar infarction
Cerebellar atrophy
Chiari malformation (Case 100)
Meningioma (Case 58)
Binswanger's disease/multiple infarcts (Case 91)
Glomus jugulare (Case 38)
Epidermoid (Case 33)
Brainstem haemorrhage (Case 68)
Subarachnoid haemorrhage (Case 13)
Multiple sclerosis (Case 70)
Arteritis (Case 27)
Arterial spasm (Case 26)
Encephalitis (Case 15)
Granulomas (Case 12)
Metastases (Cases 3 and 43)
Cerebellar astrocytoma (Case 6)
Meningitis (Case 20)
Cerebral abscess (Case 17)
Normal pressure hydrocephalus (Case 90)
Spinocerebellar degeneration
Cerebellar haemorrhage (Case 16)

Case 77

Male, aged 44 years.
Two-year history of right-sided tinnitus and deafness.

Q: The patient was investigated using two imaging
   techniques (images A, B and C). What are the
   techniques and what do they show?

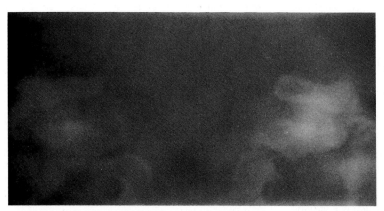

A

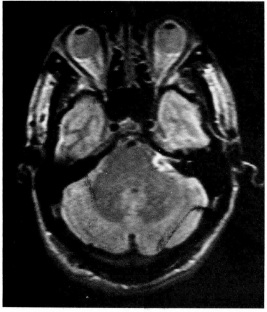

B

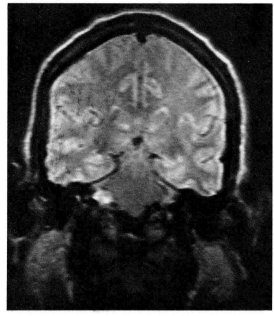

C

Case 77   Acoustic neuroma (Schwannoma)

Image A is a plain-film tomographic 'slice' in the coronal plane through the petrous bones at the level of the internal auditory canals. The canal on the left is of normal size and shape; that on the right is widened and 'trumpet-shaped'. This appearance is very suggestive of acoustic neuroma. Images B and C are T2-weighted spin-echo MRI scans in the axial and coronal plane respectively. These show a high-signal (i.e., long T2 relaxation) lesion in the right cerebello-pontine angle (CPA). A thin streak of high signal can be seen extending laterally from this lesion into the internal auditory canal area. These appearances are also consistent with the diagnosis of acoustic neuroma.

Acoustic neuroma is a common benign tumour arising from the nerve sheath of the VIIIth cranial nerve. Histologically it is more correctly described as a Schwannoma. Most of these tumours arise within the internal auditory canal, causing it to enlarge, and grow out into the CPA to produce a local mass effect. This lesion causes tinnitus, deafness and vertigo by virtue of its compression of the VIIIth nerve. If the adjacent VIIth nerve is also compressed there may be an associated facial paralysis. The larger tumours displace the brainstem and fourth ventricle. Hydrocephalus is commonly present. Imaging techniques should be reserved for those patients in whom caloric tests are positive.

Conventional CT scanning usually demonstrates the larger lesions if contrast medium is given. These tumours are often isodense with brain and can be difficult to see on the plain scan. Moderate enhancement after i.v. contrast injection is invariably present and should be given if this diagnosis is suspected (*see* image D below). These tumours lie in the CPA where they have a narrow attachment to bone (unlike meningiomas in this area which have a broader attachment). They show a uniform texture but occasionally lower density areas, probably necrotic, are present. Calcification is very unusual. Small tumours may be wholly or principally intracanalicular and these lesions may be impossible to detect on CT without air or contrast medium in the CPA to outline them. In recent years conventional tomography has fallen into disuse and CT has become the method of choice for assessment of these cases. High-resolution studies will also demonstrate the canalicular widening and indicate intrathecal studies where the canal changes are the only ones present. Angiography will show displacement of local vessels and perhaps a tumour blush in larger lesions; it has little role in management.

Many workers believe that MRI will soon become the technique of choice for the demonstration of this tumour. As in the case illustrated here, it can clearly demonstrate the intracanalicular portions of this tumour. Long T1 (low signal on inversion recovery) and long T2 (this case) are the usual pattern. Experience to date suggests that it can detect most of the wholly intracanalicular lesions without the need for intrathecal contrast agents. Gadolinium given intravenously will cause most of these lesions to enhance on MRI. The absence of bone artefact and the multi-planar capacity of MRI give it further advantages over CT. Bone deformity is not shown however.

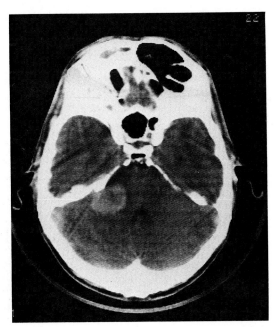

D [+C]

Case 78

Male, aged 20 years.
Diplopia, dysphagia and limb weakness for 8 months.

Q: What pulse sequences have been used for these
    MRI scans, and what lesion is demonstrated?

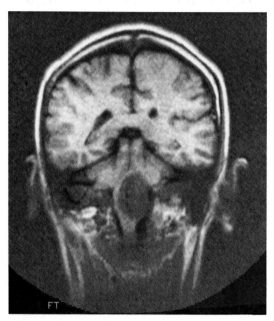

A

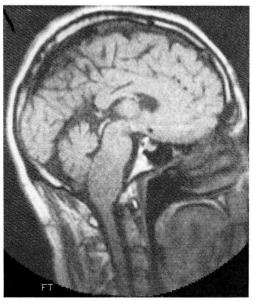

B

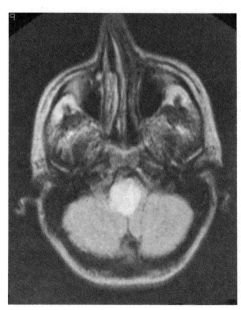

C

Case 78   Brainstem glioma

Scan A is an inversion recovery sequence image taken in the coronal plane. Anatomical detail is good and the grey matter is shown as a grey tone and white matter as white, while CSF is black: all features of a T1-weighted sequence, in this case inversion recovery. The scan plane is through the brainstem at the level of the cerebellar peduncles. The plane passes through the tentorium and the occipital horns. An ovoid low-signal (long T1) area can be seen within the lower brainstem on the left side. The brainstem is asymmetrically enlarged by this lesion. Scan B is a T1-weighted spin-echo sequence in the sagittal plane. The CSF is again of low signal, but grey/white matter differentiation is poor. The scan plane is in the midline as the aqueduct is clearly visualized. The lower brainstem (medulla) is expanded below the level of the fourth ventricle. This expansion ends quite abruptly at the junction of the medulla with the cervical cord. The enlarged area is clearly defined from the adjacent cerebellum. Scan C is a T2-weighted spin-echo sequence in the axial plane taken low in the posterior fossa. The lesion can readily be defined as an area of high signal (long T2) occupying most of the brainstem. The appearances are those of a glioma of the brainstem.

Brainstem glioma is a tumour encountered mostly in children and young adults. Its course may be quite prolonged and many patients experience a relentlessly progressive deterioration in brainstem functions. This tumour causes a wide variety of neurological symptoms and signs depending on its location and extent. Various combinations of cranial nerve palsies and long tract signs are encountered, with respiratory depression in advanced cases.

MRI now appears to be the most sensitive technique for the demonstration of this lesion; the multiplanar facility provides excellent visualization of its local extent. In common with other tumours, brainstem gliomas exhibit long T1 and T2 relaxation times as in this case. Gadolinium enhancement may better define the tumour margins and any surrounding oedema. This tumour can be difficult to detect with CT, especially in the early stages. CT is plagued with artefacts over the brainstem and contrast enhancement is often unhelpful. A tumour in the upper brainstem is shown in image D below, where the swelling of the pons is evident. Subtle expansion or deformity of the stem may be demonstrated in some cases by opacification of the basal cisterns with intrathecal contrast medium. Angiography may show displacement of adjacent vessels; occasionally tumour circulation is identified.

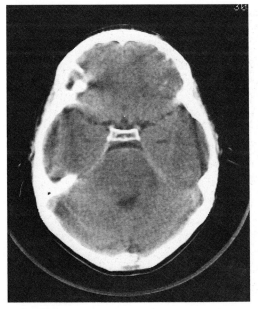

D [+C]

Case 79

Male, aged 7 years.
Five-week history of ataxia.
Recently headache and vomiting.

Q: What sort of scans are these? What do they show?

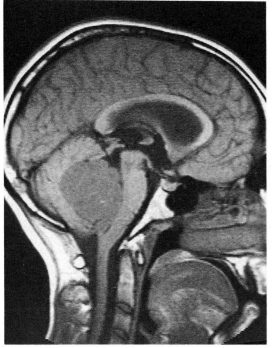

A

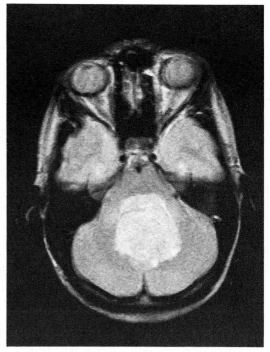

B

Case 79   Medulloblastoma

The scans are from an MRI study on this patient. Image A is a T1-weighted spin-echo sequence in the sagittal plane. This shows dilated third and lateral ventricles and a low-signal mass in the cerebellum. The T2-weighted spin-echo sequence (image B) shows the lesion to be of high intensity on this axial slice. This lesion, in common with many other tumours, presents prolonged T1 and T2 relaxation times. Biopsy revealed a medulloblastoma.

Medulloblastoma is the commonest intracranial tumour in children. Boys are more often affected than girls and the tumour may be seen in adults. It is a malignant lesion with a poor prognosis and has a distinct tendency to seed through the CSF spaces. The tumour arises in the midline and spreads through the vermis in any direction. Calcification is uncommon,

helping to differentiate it from ependymoma which is the principal differential diagnosis for tumours in this location. Choroid plexus papilloma is also found in this site but shows prominent enhancement on CT.

CT scanning shows a lesion of variable density which invariably enhances. Hydrocephalus is very common. Angiography will show non-specific signs of a tumour in this area and is of little value in management. Isotope scanning will usually show some uptake in the tumour. Gadolinium enhancement on MRI may help to define the margin of the tumour from adjacent oedema.

An enhanced CT scan on another child showing the huge enhancing mass and dilated temporal horns is shown below (image C).

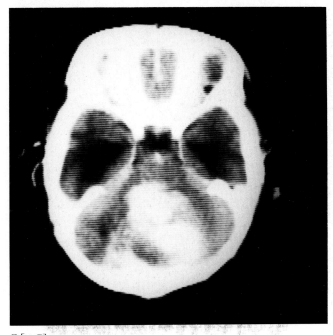

C [+C]

Case 80

Male, aged 66 years.
Three-month history of dizziness and vomiting with
headaches.

Q: These plain and enhanced CT scans were
obtained. The most likely diagnosis is:

    i   Choroid plexus papilloma.
    ii Intraventricular meningioma.
    iii Medulloblastoma.
    iv Ependymoma.

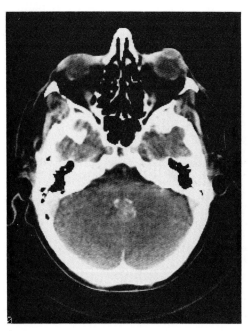

A

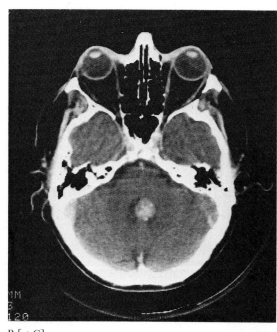

B [+C]

Case 80   Ependymoma

The plain scan shows a partly calcified lesion within the fourth ventricle. The lesion is also of generally raised density. Following enhancement the lesion shows generalized increased density. Choroid plexus papilloma is usually intraventricular and could look similar to this; it is often associated with a secretory hydrocephalus (*see* Case 42). However, it is found mostly in much younger patients. Intraventricular meningioma can show a similar appearance and would be difficult to exclude. Medulloblastoma does not usually calcify and is seen mainly in children (*see* Case 79). These appearances are due to an ependymoma.

This tumour arises from the ependymal lining of the ventricles, is commonly calcified and usually shows prominent enhancement (normally much more than this). The lesion is benign and very vascular. It may also be found in the spinal cord. Its characteristic intraventricular location often produces hydrocephalus. In children it tends to occur in the posterior fossa. In adults, a supratentorial location is more common. This diagnosis should be considered in any lesion close to or within the ventricles.

Case 81

Female, aged 59 years.
Sudden onset of severe vertigo, headaches and vomiting.

Q: What changes can be seen on these CT scans?

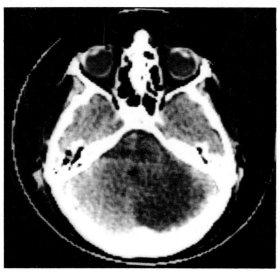

A

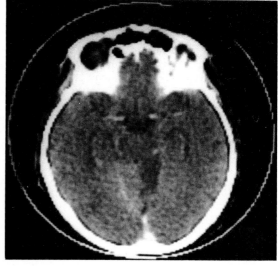

B

Case 82

Female, aged 67 years.
Increasing ataxia for 4 years.

Q: Images A and B are from a CT scan. What prominent feature is shown? What possible causes for this appearance would you consider?

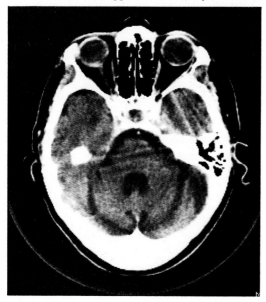

A

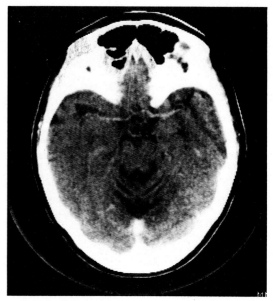

B

Case 81   Cerebellar infarction

Image A shows displacement of the fourth ventricle to the left side by an ill-defined low density in the right side of the cerebellum. Image B is taken at a slightly higher level, showing similar changes in the upper cerebellum with a sharply defined medial margin. There was no appreciable change after contrast enhancement. The sudden onset suggests a vascular event such as haemorrhage or infarction. There is no evidence of raised density to suggest haemorrhage and the appearances are consistent with acute infarction in the territory of the superior cerebellar artery. Low-density tumours or cysts could look like this but the sudden onset of symptoms is not consistent with those possibilities.

Infarction in the cerebellum is most commonly due to ischaemia in the territory of the posterior inferior cerebellar artery. Such infarcts, however, are often difficult to diagnose with certainty on CT, partly because of their low position in an area of the posterior fossa most prone to artefacts. Infarcts in the territory of the superior cerebellar artery are more readily visualized and show appearances similar to those illustrated. Midline shift is fairly common and hydrocephalus may ensue. A sharp medial margin to the lesion in the midline of the upper vermis is characteristic. Enhancement may be seen over the surface. CT provides valuable management information by conforming the diagnosis and excluding haemorrhage. Demonstration of hydrocephalus may be crucial to a patient's survival. Coexistent brainstem infarction is common but often difficult to see on CT. MRI may be superior to CT in the assessment of these cases. Angiography may be required if surgical correction of diseased arteries is contemplated.

Case 82   Cerebellar atrophy

Image A shows the patient to be somewhat asymmetrically aligned in the scanner with unequal visualization of the petrous bones. The fourth ventricle is large and there is widening of the basal cisterns around the brainstem and cerebellum. Image B is taken through the suprasellar cistern and upper vermis. The latter structure shows prominent folia with wide CSF spaces between them. The appearances are those of cerebellar atrophy.

This condition is less common than atrophy of the cerebral hemispheres (*see* Case 89) and may occur without cerebral atrophy. Ataxia and other cerebellar signs are usually present and many cases are associated with alcoholism, as in this patient.

Case 83

Female, aged 32 years.
Sudden onset of painful right IIIrd nerve palsy.

Q: A CT scan was normal. Why was this angiogram
    obtained, and what does it show?

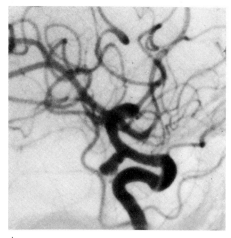

A

Case 84

Female, aged 55 years.
Four-year history of right-sided facial pain and
numbness.

Q: This base view of the skull shows gross smooth
    erosion of the right petrous apex. The most likely
    diagnosis is?

    i   Metastases.
    ii   Acoustic neuroma.
    iii Meningioma.
    iv   Glomus jugulare.
    v   Trigeminal neuroma.

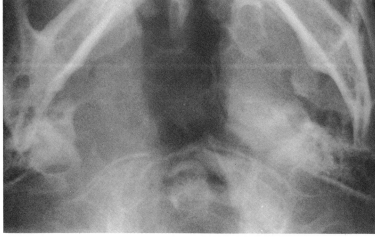

A

Case 83   Aneurysm

A painful ocular palsy of gradual or sudden onset may be due to an aneurysm in or close to the cavernous sinus pressing on the IIIrd, IVth or VIth cranial nerves. These lesions are often not sufficiently large to be seen on CT, even with enhancement, and angiography is usually necessary to exclude this possibility. The angiogram shown (image A) is of the right carotid territory. This shows a 1-cm aneurysm

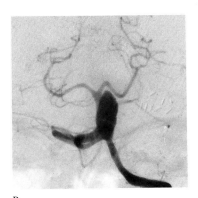

B

pointing backwards and downwards. It is seen to arise from that part of the carotid siphon just above the pituitary fossa at the level of the posterior communicating artery (although this vessel is not filled on this film). Presumably the aneurysm is pressing down on the posterior part of the IIIrd nerve.

A further example of an aneurysm causing a cranial nerve palsy is shown below in image B. This lesion arises from the posterior inferior cerebellar artery and is demonstrated on this AP vertebral artery study. The aneurysm was considerably larger than this on CT because of thrombus occluding part of its lumen. It presented with nerve deafness and diminished Vth nerve sensation.

Case 84   Trigeminal neuroma (Schwannoma)

The most likely diagnosis is a trigeminal neuroma. Metastases cause irregular destruction of bone, not a sharply marginated defect such as this, and the history is too long also. Acoustic neuroma arises more posteriorly along the petrous bone and a meningioma should produce some bone sclerosis even when the principal bone effect is erosive. Glomus jugulare tumours occur more inferiorly in the petrous bone and do not usually cause Vth nerve symptoms.

Trigeminal neuroma is an uncommon benign tumour arising from the nerve sheath. The sensory disturbance is appropriate to a Vth nerve lesion. These

lesions may present when quite small and if the mandibular division is involved the foramen ovale should be enlarged. Small lesions elsewhere along the course of the nerve may not be evident on conventional CT, and contrast medium in the CSF may be required (see Figure 96). The conventionally enhanced CT scan on this patient is shown below (image B), where the considerable size of the lesion is shown. A defect in the temporal bone is due to surgery. This degree of enhancement is unusual in neuromas. MRI may prove to be the best technique for demonstrating these lesions, especially while they are still small.

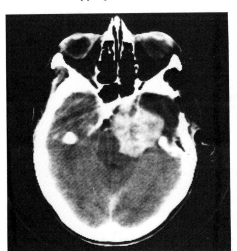

B [+C]

Case 85

Female, aged 60 years.
Sudden onset of marked cranial nerve deficits with
deteriorating conscious level.

Q: A CT scan was negative. What diagnosis can be
made from this T2-weighted MRI scan?

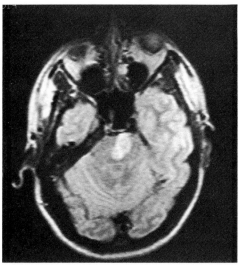

Case 86

Male, aged 30 years.
Headaches, nausea and vertigo for 2 months.

Q: These CT scans suggest which of the following
diagnoses?

    i Astrocytoma of cerebellum.
    ii Cerebellar infarction.
    iii Cerebellar abscess.
    iv Haemangioblastoma.

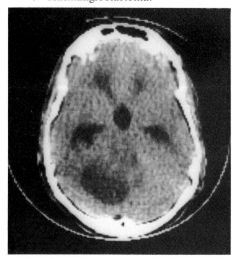

A   B [+C]

Case 85   Brainstem infarction

This axial scan shows an area of long T2 (high signal) in the anterior portion of the brainstem. The appearance is non-specific and could be due to a tumour, haemorrhage or infarct. The characteristically sudden onset suggests a haemorrhage or infarct, a T1-weighted sequence would have shown an area of low signal. A CT scan should have shown a haemorrhage, but infarcts are often very difficult to see on CT due to artefacts over the brainstem on posterior fossa slices. These lesions are usually the result of atheroma or thrombosis in the vertebrobasilar arterial system. Quite small infarcts can produce devastating clinical deficits and death often ensues.

Case 86   Haemangioblastoma

Image A (unenhanced) shows a large cystic area in the upper left cerebellar hemisphere. The ventricles are dilated. After enhancement, image B shows a densely enhancing nodule in the anterior part of the cyst. Cerebellar infarction would not show an area of this low a density, and nodular enhancement would also be atypical. Cerebellar abscess should show ring enhancement (see Case 17). Astrocytoma in the cerebellum could look like this, but a discrete nodule of enhancement would be unusual in this condition which tends to occur in a younger age-group than this.

Haemangioblastoma is an uncommon benign tumour which usually presents as a vascular nodule in the wall of a cyst. The lesion tends to occur in middle life, and lies laterally in the cerebellar hemisphere. Angiography shows a characteristically highly vascular nodule, and these may be multiple. The lesion may be associated with multiple retinal tumours (von Hippel–Lindau's syndrome).

Case 87

Female, aged 19 years.
Seven-month history of complete left VIth nerve and partial left IIIrd nerve palsies.

Q: This sagittal tomogram shows a normal odontoid peg inferiorly, and an area of vague calcification and destruction of the clivus extending up into the pituitary fossa (partly destroyed). A soft tissue mass extends into the nasopharynx. The most likely diagnosis is?

i   Chordoma.
ii Meningioma.
iii Paget's disease.
iv Metastatic deposit.

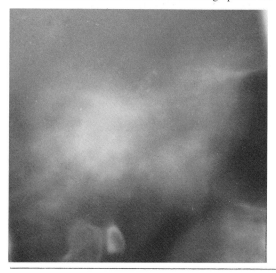

Case 88

Female, aged 68 years.
Five-year history of headaches, bulbar palsies and intellectual loss.

Q: What generalized disease process and anatomical derangement are shown on this film?

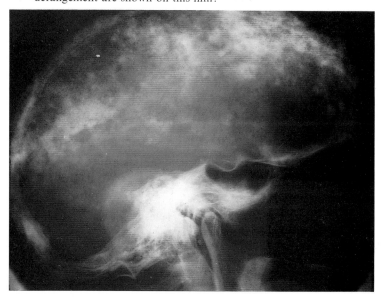

Case 87   Chordoma of the clivus

The most likely diagnosis is a chordoma of the clivus. This tumour is relatively benign and occurs mostly in the clivus or sacrum. The characteristic appearance is of prominent calcification and destruction of the clivus and adjacent bones. CT scanning will show similar appearances with variable enhancement. MRI scanning will show the tumour mass but the bone destruction and calcification may be masked on this technique. The lesion is usually in the midline and since it can arise in a high or low position on the clivus a variety of clinical presentations may be seen, including headache, raised intracranial pressure and cranial nerve palsies.

Other lesions arise in this position. Meningioma would rarely be this extensive or destructive. Paget's disease shows thickening of bone rather than calcification and destruction. Metastatic deposits are seen in this location but rarely show calcification.

Case 88   Paget's disease of the skull/basilar invagination

This lateral skull film shows mottled density throughout the vault. This could be due to metastatic disease, but the texture of the bone is generally abnormal and the density changes are too fine. The pattern is that of Paget's disease of the skull. This condition, of unknown aetiology, is found in older patients and causes thickening and softening of the bones. The skull base or vault may be affected. Vault involvement may be of increased or decreased bone density. This may produce headaches. Lesions in the skull base may cause more neurological disturbance because of narrowing of the foraminae and compromise of the cranial nerves. Marked softening of the skull base may lead to 'basilar invagination'. This is a deformity in which the cranio-cervical junction is displaced upwards into the skull base. In a normal situation a line drawn from the posterior margin of the hard palate to the posterior margin of the foramen magnum will pass above or just through the tip of the odontoid peg. When basilar invagination is present most of the odontoid peg is above the line (Chamberlain's line—*see* Case 96). The resulting distortion of the clivus, brainstem and cranial nerves produces a variety of symptoms. Hydrocephalus may be present as well. Basilar invagination may also be the result of rickets, developmental disorders, etc.

Dementia and psychotic states

General considerations

This chapter is concerned with disorders of the mind. The majority of psychotic and neurotic disorders are not usually the concern of neuroradiology; however, psychotic states where the presenting features suggest an underlying organic cause may be worthy of further investigation. In summary, patients with associated neurological symptoms or signs, or those whose mental state has deteriorated steadily over a short period, are certainly worthy of further assessment.

The term dementia is generally applied to a diffuse loss of intellectual functions. Certain parameters of these functions may be particularly involved, such as memory, motivation, judgement, perception, orientation, etc. Often several modalities are simultaneously involved, although to varying degrees. The pattern of cognitive impairment, mode of onset and progression often gives a clue about the pathological process and anatomical site of the lesion. Frontal involvement is found in tertiary syphilis and Pick's disease, while Alzheimer's disease produces a temporoparietal pattern of involvement. A certain degree of such intellectual loss seems inevitable with advancing age. It is important to distinguish this condition from depression or schizophrenia. In these latter conditions detachment or apathy may lead the examiner to believe that dementia is the fundamental cause.

In later life most cases of dementia are due to the apparently inevitable processes of brain ageing. When such changes are evident before the age of 60, 'presenile dementia' is said to be present. The most common cause of this is probably Alzheimer's disease. Beyond the age of 65, the term 'senile dementia' is used for those cases where no identifiable cause is established. At least some of these will have resulted from some form of chronic ischaemic process resulting in Binswanger's disease (subcortical arteriosclerotic encephalopathy), or in the less clear-cut 'multi-infarct' dementia.

There are, however, a number of other possible causes of dementia and it is important to realize that some of these are potentially correctable. Alcoholism or other exposure to toxins or deficiencies should always be excluded. Endocrine or vitamin deficiencies, anaemia and metabolic disorders can be excluded by a detailed history and blood tests. In the rest, a case can be made for imaging investigations in patients who have had dementia for more than 1 month or less than 1 year. Partially selected series of such patients may show up to 10 per cent 'treatable lesions' on imaging techniques. However, since a proportion of these 'treatable lesions' will be high-grade gliomas or metastases, the eventual outcome is unsatisfactory. Nevertheless, a significant proportion of patients will show hydrocephalus, subdural haematomas or benign tumours—all potentially curable.

CT has been the mainstay of the investigation of dementia for many years. Most of the structural lesions that can cause dementia are readily demonstrated by this technique; other imaging studies apart from plain skull films are rarely required. Where CT is not available nuclear medicine studies will help to exclude the major correctable causes of dementia apart from hydrocephalus. MRI provides a great deal of information about grey and white matter not readily available by other studies, and this capacity, together with anticipated spectroscopic information, could greatly improve our understanding of dementia in years to come.

The pathological processes which may be associated with dementia and have imaging manifestations are listed below. Psychiatric presentations may be seen in most of these conditions.

Cerebral atrophy
Cerebellar atrophy (Case 82)
Hydrocephalus
Cerebral ischaemia/multi-infarct/Binswanger's
  disease
Chronic subdural haematoma
Intracranial tumours
Cerebral infection or granuloma (Cases 12 and 17)
Leucodystrophy (Case 34)
Previous cerebral trauma
Parkinson's disease
Huntington's disease
Jakob–Creutzfeldt disease
Pick's disease
Tertiary syphilis

Case 89

Male, aged 68 years.
Progressive disorientation, confusion and intellectual
loss over 3 years.

Q: What generalized abnormality is shown on this
    patient's CT scans?

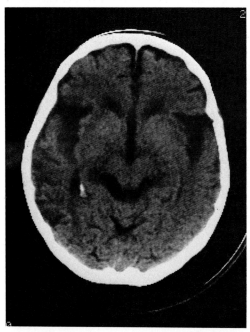

A

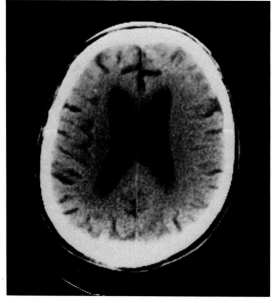

B

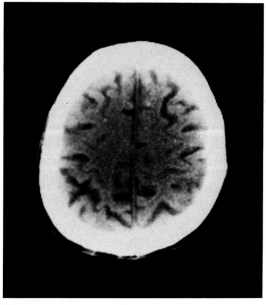

C

Case 89   Cerebral atrophy

These three CT scans are unenhanced and show generalized widening of the cortical sulci. The Sylvian and interhemispheral fissures are also enlarged; the ventricles are dilated. The appearances are those of marked cerebral atrophy.

Cerebral atrophy is a general term applied to loss of brain substance. This may be focal and result from trauma, radiation, etc. Generalized loss of neural tissue is a consequence of various degenerative disorders, including Alzheimer's, Huntington's and Jakob–Creutzfeldt diseases. Normal ageing also may result in a slow progressive brain atrophy. These generalized, degenerative processes cause loss of volume of neural tissue. This in turn is reflected by increased volume of the CSF spaces which enlarge to take up the additional space left by the shrinking brain. It is this increase in the size of the subarachnoid and ventricular compartments that produces the changes visible on the CT scans. It has been shown, however, that the degree of sulcal widening correlates poorly with the intellectual loss, although it seems that ventricular dilatation may provide a marginally closer relationship. In practice, the purpose of CT scanning is to exclude other treatable causes of dementia; but the finding of a degree of atrophy, such as is demonstrated here, is too excessive to be normal in a patient of this age.

The most important differential diagnosis of this condition is hydrocephalus. In both, the ventricles are dilated. Hydrocephalus may show interstitial oedema or periventricular flare (*see* Case 6). This feature is not seen in atrophy. Also, the ventricles tend to be bigger in hydrocephalus but temporal horn dilatation is not a prominent feature of atrophy. In atrophy the angle between the frontal horns is flatter than the more acute angle seen in hydrocephalus. Patients with hydrocephalus show ventricles that are disproportionately large for any sulcal widening that may be present due to normal ageing. The principles for differentiating these conditions are further discussed in Case 90.

Huntington's chorea may show specific atrophy of the caudate nuclei, but this sign is not a constant feature, even in advanced cases. Atrophy of the cerebellar structures is often unimpressive in cases of cerebral atrophy. Furthermore, this type of atrophy often occurs in isolation; it is discussed in Case 82.

Case 90

Male, aged 60 years.
Progressive dementia for 6 months.
Mild ataxia.

Q: Images A and B are from a CT scan on this patient. What possible diagnoses would you consider?

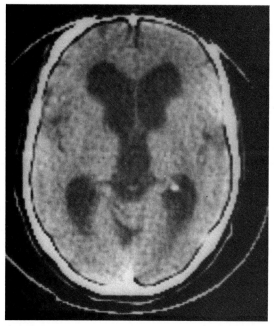

A

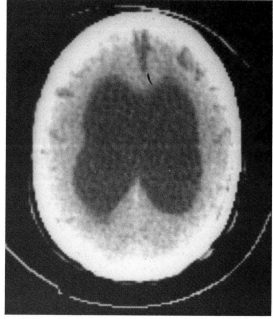

B

Case 90 Communicating hydrocephalus ('normal-pressure')

Scans A and B show marked dilatation of the third and lateral ventricles. The fourth ventricle was mildly dilated on lower slices. There is widening of the cortical sulci. The differential diagnosis here lies between cerebral atrophy and communicating hydrocephalus. Patients with atrophy usually show ventricular dilatation in proportion to the degree of sulcal widening. In the present case the ventricular dilatation does seem out of proportion to the width of sulci over the cortex. Acute hydrocephalus usually shows dark, low-density areas in the white matter around the frontal horns. This 'flare' is seen where the hydrocephalus is of recent onset, e.g., tumours, haemorrhage, etc., and is probably the result of periventricular interstitial oedema due to altered transependymal CSF resorption (see Case 6). It may be seen in established communicating hydrocephalus but is not evident in this case. When present it is a useful pointer to the cause being hydrocephalus rather than atrophy but similar appearances may be seen with deep ischaemia. Recent work with MRI suggests that this technique may help in delineating these processes. Other useful differentiating features include dilated temporal horns and an acute angle between the frontal horns (see Case 89), however the differentiation of these two conditions can be very difficult.

Communicating hydrocephalus is an important cause of dementia. For a further description of the likely causes and classification of this condition see

Case 63. In older patients it often presents with dementia and may be of the 'normal-pressure' type. The classic description of normal-pressure hydrocephalus comprises a patient with dementia, ataxia, incontinence and in whom there is evidence of hydrocephalus with normal pressure levels. In practice these patients show waves of increased pressure on intracranial monitoring and many believe this may be the best method of distinguishing those demented patients most likely to benefit from shunting. In cases where doubt exists it has been customary to confirm the presence of CSF pathway obstruction by studying the patterns of CSF flow. This may be done using isotope or contrast medium in the CSF. In both cases the marker may enter the ventricles during the first 12–18 hours after lumbar injection, but should be cleared from the ventricles by 24 hours in normal patients. The pattern of flow in the basal cisterns may also be helpful. This technique was performed on this patient and the scans are shown below. Image C was taken 6 hours after the injection and shows that contrast medium has entered the ventricles. At 36 hours some clearing has occurred (image D) but the ventricles are still more dense than on the precontrast scans A and B. There is evidence, therefore, of delayed clearing of contrast medium from the ventricles, indicating communicating hydrocephalus. The patient was shunted and there was significant improvement in his clinical condition.

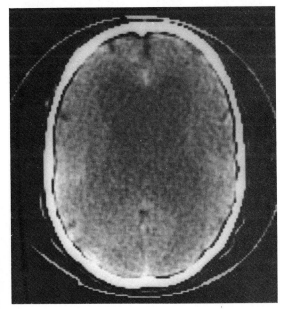

C

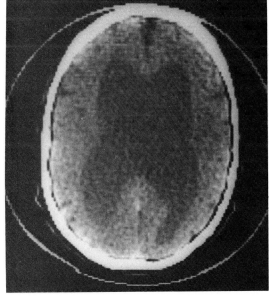

D

Case 91

Male, aged 71 years.
Psychosis with increasing dementia for 14 months.

Q: These CT scans were obtained. There was no change after contrast enhancement. Which of these diagnoses would you consider?

   i   Cerebral atrophy.
   ii Metastatic disease.
   iii Leucodystrophy.
   iv Subcortical arteriosclerotic encephalopathy.

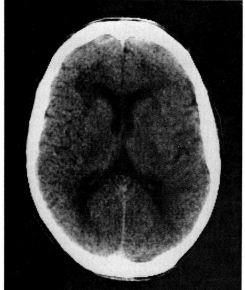
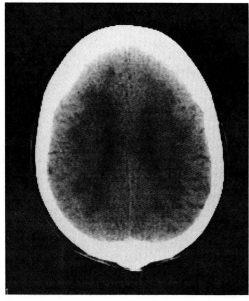

A   B

Case 91   Subcortical arteriosclerotic encephalopathy/multi-infarct dementia

These scans show symmetrical low-density areas adjacent to the frontal horns and the posterior lateral ventricles. The lesions are adjacent to the ependymal lining of the ventricles. Similar densities may be seen in recent hydrocephalus due to transependymal resorption of CSF, but in hydrocephalus the frontal low densities are more anteriorly placed. There is no evidence of ventricular dilatation in this case. There is no dilatation of cortical sulci or fissures to suggest cerebral atrophy. Metastatic deposits invariably show areas of enhancement and their associated oedema would not be this symmetrical. Leucodystrophy could look like this, but at this age one would expect an identifiable cause such as cytotoxic drugs. The findings are consistent with subcortical arteriosclerotic encephalopathy.

This condition, also known as Binswanger's disease, is increasingly being recognized as an important cause of dementia. The appearances on CT represent areas of myelin and axon loss. The changes are related to sclerosis of arterioles in the white matter. Hypertension appears to play a major role in causation in many patients. Some patients show associated ventricular dilatation.

The relationship between this condition and 'multiple-infarct' dementia is unclear. Some patients with progressive dementia have CT scans showing several focal cortical infarcts. These are wedge-shaped lesions in typical arterial territory distribution. Small deep lacunar infarcts may also be associated. Unlike subcortical arteriosclerotic encephalopathy, the cortical lesions are not confined to the white matter and extend to the brain surface. Affected patients may give a history of incremental deterioration. An example of this is illustrated below in C.

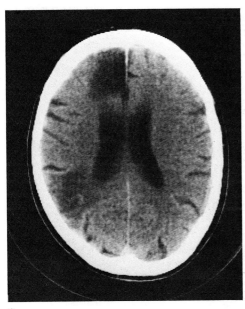

C

Case 92

Male, aged 74 years.
Five-week history of increasing confusion and disorientation.
Mild right-sided weakness.

Q: This frontal view of an isotope brain scan shows an area of increased uptake over the upper left hemisphere. The most likely diagnosis is?

    i   Meningioma.
    ii Infarction.
    iii Subdural haematoma.
    iv Cerebral atrophy.

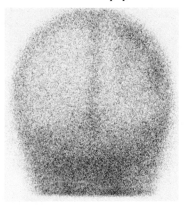

Case 93

Female, aged 67 years.
Intellectual loss for 6 months.
Some headaches and right-sided weakness.

Q: These CT scans suggest which diagnosis?

    i   Cerebral lymphoma.
    ii Meningioma.
    iii Aneurysm.
    iv Glioma.
    v   Metastatic deposit.

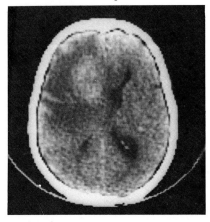

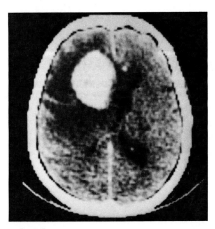

A   B [+C]

Case 92   Chronic subdural haematoma

Meningioma may be found in this location but usually shows prominent uptake and tends to be more localized. The uptake here is diffuse over the upper hemisphere, unlike infarction where the pattern tends to be more localized and wedge-shaped. Cerebral atrophy or Alzheimer's disease do not show any focal abnormality on isotope studies. This uptake pattern is typical of a chronic subdural haematoma. This pathological process is described in Cases 7 and 32, and covers a significant portion of the hemisphere at the time of injury. As the capsule develops the resorbing haematoma becomes more contained. The haematoma and its local effects may cause increased uptake at quite an early stage and this technique can be helpful in excluding this important cause of dementia where CT scanning is not available.

Case 93   Primary lymphoma of brain (microglioma)

The plain scan (A) shows an ill-defined raised density area deep in the left frontal lobe with extensive surrounding oedema and mass effect. Scan B shows dense enhancement within the lesion. All of the suggested diagnoses are possible here and a conclusive diagnosis cannot be made from this study alone. Biopsy was performed revealing a primary cerebral lymphoma. This condition, which used to be called microglioma, is an important diagnosis to suspect, since many patients respond very well to radiotherapy. In many respects the CT appearances are similar to meningioma but the lesion is less well-defined and the enhancement is usually more striking. The lesion may spread along the margins of the ventricle and look like ventriculitis (see Case 17).

Case 94

Male, aged 73 years.
Increasing confusion and disorientation for 6 weeks.

Q: This enhanced CT scan was obtained. The most
likely diagnosis is?

    i   Metastases.
    ii Cerebral abscess.
    iii Cerebral tuberculosis.
    iv Malignant glioma.

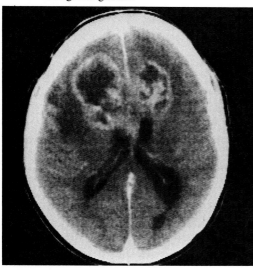

[+C]

Case 95

Male, aged 38 years.
Long history of schizophrenia.
Recent deterioration.

Q: What surgical procedure has been performed on
this patient?

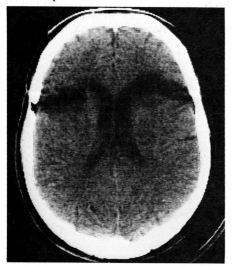

Case 94   Glioma of the corpus callosum

The irregularly outlined enhancing ring areas in both frontal lobes are joined by a bridge of abnormal (enhancing) tissue across the anterior corpus callosum. The enhancing rings are too irregular in outline and wall thickness to be abscesses. Metastases could look like this but do not usually grow to this size while a patient still survives. The granulomas of cerebral tuberculosis could exhibit this appearance, but in this form they are very unusual outside areas where TB is endemic.

Tumours in the corpus callosum commonly present with dementia-like syndromes as a result of disturbance of the communicating fibres passing between the hemispheres. Consequently, lesions in this site should be considered in such patients. However, many of them will show neurological signs to suggest the presence of a focal lesion.

Case 95   Bifrontal leucotomy

This unenhanced CT-scan slice through the lateral ventricles shows symmetrical low-density bands running through the region just behind the frontoparietal junction. The position and appearance of these lesions is quite unlike anything occurring naturally and they are 'man-made'. A small defect is seen in the vault on the left side adjacent to the most lateral part of the band on that side. A similar defect was present on the right-hand side on another slice.

These bone defects are due to burr holes; the patient had previously undergone the operation of 'bifrontal leucotomy'. This procedure is now rarely performed, but was used to alleviate longstanding psychiatric disorders in some patients. This patient had received some benefit from this technique many years before. During the operation, fibres in the frontoparietal area were cut, leaving these appearances on the CT scan.

Congenital lesions

General considerations

Congenital abnormalities of the brain, skull and spinal cord are common and very varied. Several examples have already been discussed in earlier sections of this book. In this section, however, a very simplified summary of congenital lesions of the brain is given. Some further examples are shown on the pages which follow.

Broadly speaking these congenital abnormalities can be grouped as follows:

1. Neural tube defects: these include meningoceles, encephaloceles and the Chiari malformation.
2. Disorganization of the cerebral hemispheres: this refers principally to corpus callosum defects and holoprosencephaly.
3. Dysplasia of the cerebral cortex: primarily producing abnormal migration of neurones, this group comprises the variants of agyria (lissencephaly) and schizencephaly.
4. Destructive lesions such as porencephaly and hydranencephaly.
5. The phakomatoses: this genetically transmitted group includes tuberous sclerosis, Sturge–Weber disease and the many forms of neurofibromatosis.

The causes of congenital abnormalities are many and most conditions are poorly understood. Exposure to ionizing radiation, drugs or infectious diseases may play a part in some cases. In most instances, however, a cause is not established but associated abnormalities elsewhere in the body are not uncommon. The point in time during the development of the fetus when these abnormalities occur is variable, ranging from as little as 4 weeks in severe holoprosencephaly, to very much later for some of the other lesions.

Some of these conditions may be obvious at birth by virtue of the child's physical appearance, e.g., encephalocele. Others may only become manifest later when retardation of normal development is apparent. Lesions such as the phakomatoses may go unnoticed until adult life.

Imaging investigations can usually be confined to plain films of the skull and CT scanning. The former shows the general shape of the skull and possible bone defects; calcification or abnormalities at the cranio-vertebral junction. CT scanning will usually provide sufficient anatomical detail to permit a diagnosis in most cases. MRI may be helpful in some lesions such as the Chiari malformation. Angiography may show the position of important vessels if corrective surgery is planned for lesions such as an encephalocele.

Some congenital lesions affecting the skull are shown in Part I. The congenital lesions discussed in Part II are listed below.

Basilar invagination/assimilation
Encephalocele
Dandy–Walker syndrome
Chiari malformation
Dysgenesis of corpus callosum
Arachnoid cysts (Case 44)
Porencephaly (Case 45)
Aqueduct stenosis (Case 5)
Tuberous sclerosis (Case 53)
Sturge–Weber syndrome (Case 54)
Neurofibromatosis (Case 10)

Case 96

Male, aged 26 years.
Increasing weakness of limbs over several years.
Some cranial nerve palsies.

Q: What diagnostic techniques are these, and what
      pathology is shown?

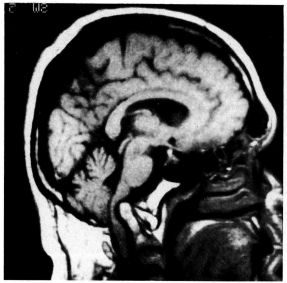

A

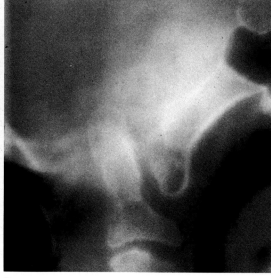

B

Case 96   Basilar invagination with congenital craniocervical assimilation

Image A is a T1-weighted MRI scan in the sagittal plane. The lower brainstem is focally displaced and indented by a displaced odontoid peg. In front of the peg and at the lower end of the clivus is seen a further high-signal (short T1) triangular structure 'pointing' upwards and backwards. This is a deformed anterior arch of atlas fused to the lower clivus. These three structures (odontoid, clivus and arch of atlas) are all high-signal on this sequence. This is not because they are bony, but as a result of their marrow content (marrow has a high lipid content and lipid has a short T1). The appearances are those of compression of the brainstem by basilar invagination. In this condition there is inversion or invagination of the margins of the foramen magnum, i.e., clivus and lower edge of occipital bone, allowing upward movement of the odontoid peg. This anatomical distortion may be the result of a congenital abnormality, as in this case, but frequently follows softening of the skull base by bone

diseases such as Paget's disease (*see* Case 88). In this case the deformity is associated with congenital assimilation of the atlas. This situation is a fusion (partial or complete) of the atlas (C1) to the margins of the foramen magnum. Such assimilation is associated with the Arnold–Chiari malformation in a significant number of cases (*see* Case 100).

Image B is a sagittal tomograph on this patient and shows the bony structures also demonstrated on the MRI scan. The abnormally large anterior arch of the atlas can be seen to be fused to the lower clivus. The posterior arch is completely absorbed into the posterior lip of the foramen magnum.

The presence of basilar invagination in mild cases can be confirmed by Chamberlain's line. This runs from the posterior margin of the hard palate to the posterior margin of the foramen magnum. Normally not more than 2 mm of the odontoid peg lies above this line (*see* image C).

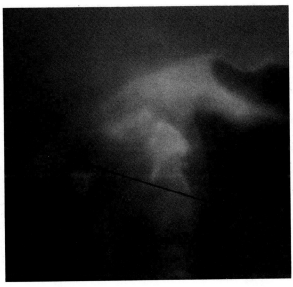

C

Case 97

Female, aged 19 months.
Bulge above nasal bridge (between eyes) since birth.

Q: The PA film of the skull shows a bony deformity.
   What is your diagnosis?

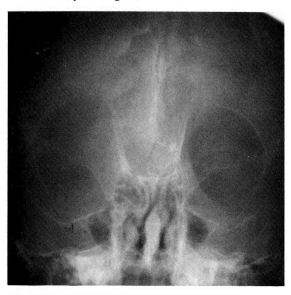

Case 98

Male, aged 3 months.
Increasing head circumference since birth.

Q: These CT scans are typical of what diagnosis?

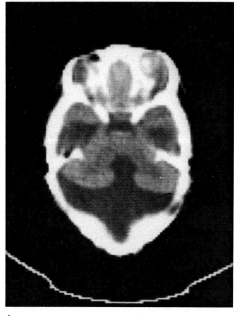

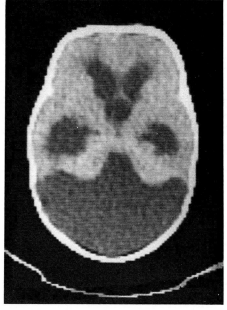

A   B

Case 97   Encephalocele

The plain skull film shows separation of the orbits (hypertelorism) by a bone defect in the midline of the frontal bone. This was directly underneath the palpable lump and the appearances are typical of an encephalocele. This lesion is a congenital herniation of brain, with a covering of meninges, through a defect in the vault. These are most common in the occipital area, but are found elsewhere including the base, where they may present as masses in the nasal cavity. Herniation containing meninges only are called meningoceles. The bone defect may be very small in relation to the size of the herniation. CT scans may help to confirm that brain tissue is present within such a lesion. Associated abnormalities such as corpus callosum defects may also be present.

Case 98   Dandy–Walker syndrome

Image A shows a dilated fourth ventricle communicating with a large cisterna magna. There is no evidence of normal vermis tissue (see Figure 70). Image B shows the abnormality extending up to the tentorium which is unusually high in position. The third and lateral ventricles are dilated. Since the fourth ventricle is dilated, the ventricular block must lie at the outlets of the fourth ventricle. In the Dandy–Walker syndrome there is congenital atresia of the outlet foramina and agenesis of the vermis. These features lead to a dilated fourth ventricle in continuity with this huge dilated space, causing expansion of the posterior fossa. This can be seen on plain films as upward displacement of the venous sinus grooves reflecting the high position of the tentorium. Mild forms of this condition exist, but should not be confused with a normal large cisterna magna or an arachnoid cyst. In these latter cases the vermis is present.

This normally can also be demonstrated readily with MRI. In the neonate an angled coronal ultrasound study may demonstrate the posterior fossa anatomy sufficiently well to allow this diagnosis to be made.

Case 99

Female, aged 15 years.
Recently two fits.
Proptosis right eye.

Q: These CT scans were obtained. The most likely
    diagnosis is?

i   Hydrocephalus.
ii Third ventricle tumour.
iii Dysgenesis of corpus callosum.

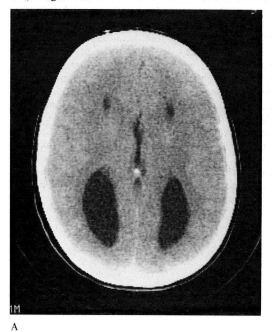

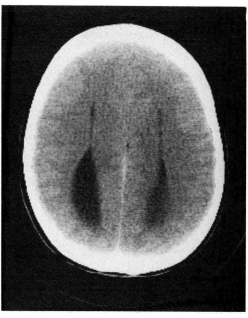

A

B

Case 100

Female, aged 20 years.
Nine-month history of limb weakness.

Q: What diagnostic technique is this? What
    abnormality is present at the cranio-vertebral
    junction?

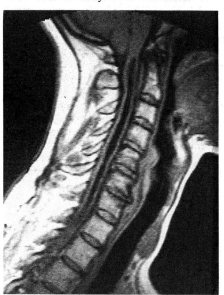

Case 99   Dysgenesis of corpus callosum

The scans show unusually wide separation of the lateral ventricles that also extend high into the hemispheric white matter. The third ventricle extends upwards between them. This appearance is due to failure of normal development of the corpus callosum, allowing the ventricles to develop in these abnormal positions. Some occipital horn dilatation is commonly present. The dysgenesis may range from partial to complete. Partial dysgenesis is usually seen posteriorly. Anterior extension allows the anterior interhemispheral fissure to extend to the anterior third ventricle. The clinical effects of this condition depend on the degree of extension. Low intelligence and fits are among the commonest manifestations.

This defect may occur in association with other abnormalities, including Dandy–Walker syndrome, holoprosencephaly, encephalocele, etc. (In this case neurofibromatosis was also present, accounting for the proptosis.) About 40 per cent of intracranial lipomas occur in association with dysgenesis of the corpus callosum. These show a characteristic appearance of fat density with curved marginal calcification in the anterior corpus callosum. The calcification may be visible in this characteristic shape on the plain PA skull film. A CT scan of such a lipoma is shown in image C.

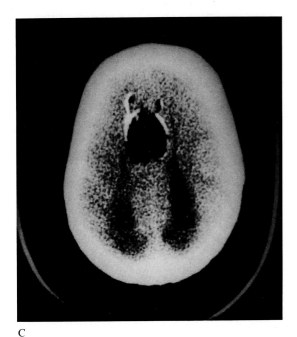

C

Case 100   Chiari I malformation and syringomyelia

This is a midline sagittal MRI scan. A T1-weighted spin-echo sequence has been used. This renders CSF of low signal that can be seen around the spinal cord. The cord itself is enlarged and contains a long low-signal lesion suggestive of a cyst, extending over many segments. At the cranio-cervical junction the cerebellar tonsils extend below the foramen magnum to the level of the arch of C1. This feature is consistent with the Chiari malformation. In this condition various degrees of abnormal position of the cerebellar tonsils are seen in this area. This case represents a Type I form. The Type II form (also known as the Arnold–Chiari malformation) shows associated downward displacement of the fourth ventricle and pons with kinking of the pontomedullary junction.

More severe forms show portions of the fourth ventricle and brainstem lying in the cervical canal. Spina bifida and meningocele are commonly associated.

The bony posterior fossa may be small and fusion of C1 to the occiput is also seen. Cystic cavitation of the spinal cord is present in many cases (syringomyelia). Presenting symptoms include cord problems or posterior fossa manifestations such as cranial nerve deficits. The bony abnormalities can be shown on plain films, especially tomography. Myelography with intrathecal enhancement can also demonstrate this area well, but the sagittal imaging and non-invasive nature of MRI make this the obvious first choice.

Suggested further reading

Du Boulay G. H. (ed) (1984) *A Textbook of Radiological Diagnosis (5th edition). Vol. I, The Head and Central Nervous System*. London: H. K. Lewis. (A comprehensive text of neuroimaging including the spine, primarily of interest to radiologists in general and to neuroradiologists in particular.)

Grainger R. G. and Allison D. J. (eds) (1986) *Diagnostic Radiology—an Anglo American Textbook of Imaging*, Vols I and III. Edinburgh: Churchill Livingstone. (A three-volume multi-author textbook of contemporary diagnostic imaging. The sections relating to the brain are of broad general interest.)

Moseley I. (1986) *Diagnostic Imaging in Neurological Disease*. Edinburgh: Churchill Livingstone. (Although primarily directed at clinicians, this should be required reading for all involved in neuroimaging. Analyses in detail the real effectiveness of traditional diagnostic imaging approaches as appraised in the literature. Reaffirms the value of much, but casts down countless myths.)

Pathology index

Index